AYURVEDA SIMPLIFIED

EMBRACING WELLNESS FOR EVERYDAY LIFE

DR. PRASANNA KAKUNJE | M. D. (AYURVEDA)

Rāgādirogān satatanuṣaktān aśeṣakāya prasrūtān aśeṣān
Autsukya moharatīdān jaghāna yo'purvavaidyāya namo'stu tasmai.

A.H.Su-1 (Vagbhata)

Sensual desire, hatred, and delusion,
The three dreadful roots of disease's infusion.
Continuously flowing, spanning lives untold,
Covering all beings, their suffering unfolds.

Restless, anxious, and deluded minds ensue,
Creating discontent, and problems anew.
To the physician who grasps this profound law,
I humbly bow, for removing disease's claw.

Contents

Connect With The Author — vii

Preface — ix

Acknowledgements — xi

1. Introduction — 1

2. The Essence Of Ayurveda — 7

3. Ayurvedic Lifestyle Principles — 21

4. Ayurvedic Nutrition — 34

5. Ayurvedic Psychology — 46

6. Ayurvedic Beauty And Self-care — 58

7. Ayurveda For Women's Health — 69

8. Ayurveda And Relationships — 80

9. Ayurveda For The Modern World — 89

10. Conclusion — 101

11. Appendix — 108

Connect With The Author

DR. PRASANNA KAKUNJE. MD(AYU)
prasanna@kakunje.com
Mobile & WhatsApp: +91 76 999 15 999
Websites:
www.ayurvedasimplified.com (Buy My Books and Read Blog Posts)
www.kakunjeayurveda.com (Ayurveda clinic)
Address:
Kakunje Publications, Kakunje Wellness,
First Floor, Janani Complex, Nagarakatte Road,
MOODUBIDRI 574227, Karnataka, India

Preface

Dear Readers,

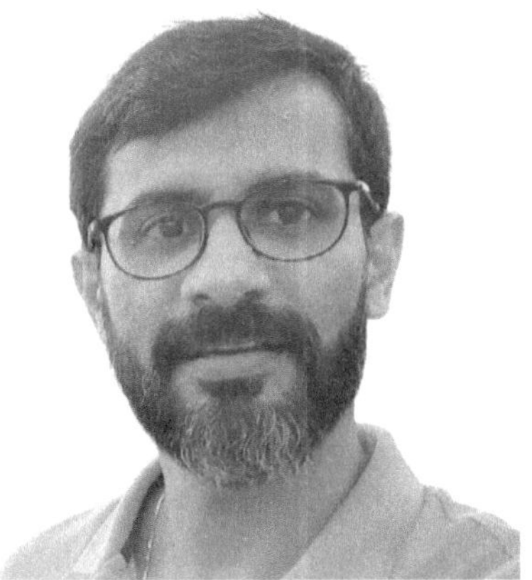

Dr. Prasanna Kakunje, MD (Ayu)

I am thrilled to present to you "Ayurveda Simplified: Embracing Wellness for Everyday Life," a book that has been crafted with a deep passion for Ayurveda and a strong desire to make its wisdom accessible to all. As an experienced Ayurvedic practitioner, it has always been my dream to distill the essence of this ancient healing tradition into simple and practical guidance that can be seamlessly integrated into your daily life.

In today's fast-paced world, where stress and health challenges are all too common, Ayurveda offers a profound and holistic approach to well-being. With its roots dating back thousands of years, Ayurveda recognizes the interconnectedness of mind, body, and spirit, and emphasizes the importance of finding balance within ourselves and in our interactions with the world around us.

In this book, I have endeavored to demystify Ayurveda and present its principles in a way that resonates with modern lifestyles. You will embark on a journey of discovery, beginning with an understanding of Ayurveda's origin and philosophy. You will learn about the three doshas - Vata, Pitta, and Kapha - and how they influence our unique constitution or Prakriti. Armed with this knowledge, you will gain insights into creating a personalized approach to wellness that aligns with your individual needs.

From lifestyle practices to nutrition, psychology, beauty, women's health, relationships, and navigating the challenges of the modern world, each chapter explores a specific aspect of Ayurveda and offers practical guidance for incorporating its wisdom into your life. You will find tips, recipes, self-assessment tools, and resources that empower you to make informed choices and embark on a journey of self-healing and self-discovery.

It is my sincere hope that this book serves as a trusted companion on your path to wellness. Whether you are new to Ayurveda or already familiar with its principles, my aim is to inspire and empower you to embrace Ayurveda as a lifelong journey of self-care, self-discovery, and vibrant well-being.

Please remember that the information provided in this book is for educational purposes and should not replace professional medical advice. If you have specific health concerns, it is important to consult with a qualified healthcare provider or Ayurvedic practitioner.

I invite you to dive in, explore, and embark on this transformative journey with Ayurveda as your guide. May this book be a beacon of light, leading you to a life of balance, vitality, and lasting wellness.

With warm regards,

Dr. Prasanna Kakunje, MD in Ayurveda

prasanna@kakunje.com

www.kakunjeayurveda.com | www.ayurvedasimplified.com

01-06-2023

Acknowledgements

"To the Brahman - Gurave Namah
To my Parents
To my Teachers
To my wife Dr. Anuradha and son Abhinav
To all the stakeholders of Ayurveda
To Life and Beyond..."

Introduction

- The journey to wellness
- Ayurveda as a holistic approach
- Overview of the book's contents

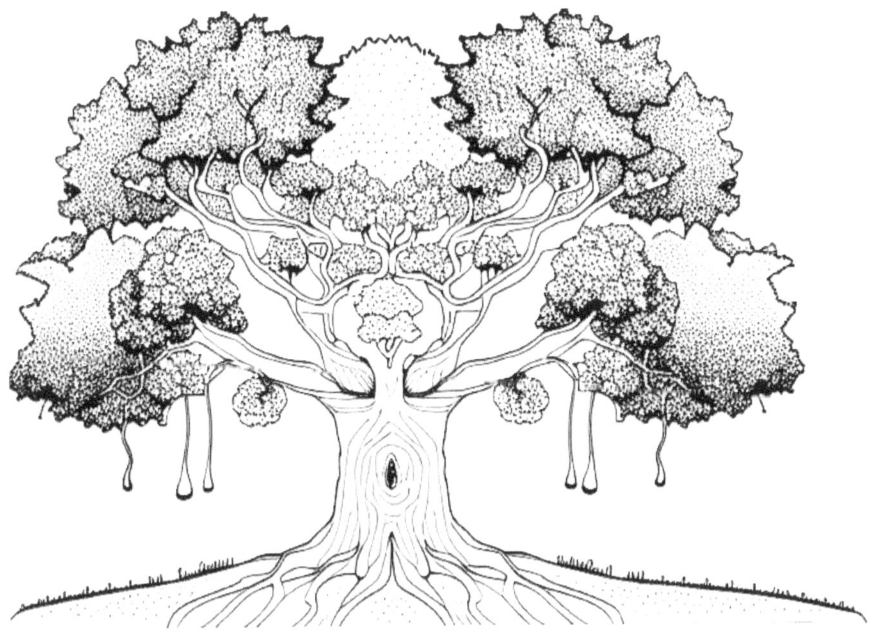

The Tree of Life

Welcome to "Ayurveda Simplified: Embracing Wellness for Everyday Life" In this comprehensive guide, we embark on a transformative journey of self-discovery and holistic wellness through the ancient wisdom of Ayurveda. Drawing inspiration from the timeless teachings of Ayurveda, we explore the profound interconnectedness of mind, body, and spirit, unveiling the keys to vibrant health, balance, and harmony.

Ayurveda, which means "the science of life," has been practiced for thousands of years in the Indian subcontinent. It offers a profound understanding of the human body and its relationship with the natural world, recognizing that we are an inseparable part of the intricate tapestry of the universe. Ayurveda empowers us to align with the rhythms of nature, awaken our innate healing potential, and lead a life filled with vitality, purpose, and joy.

In the pages that follow, we delve into the core principles of Ayurveda, providing you with a holistic roadmap to integrate its wisdom into your daily life. We begin by exploring the essence of Ayurveda, unraveling its rich philosophical foundations and unveiling the three doshas—Vata, Pitta, and Kapha—that shape our unique constitution and govern our physical, mental, and emotional well-being.

Building upon this foundation, we guide you through the practical application of Ayurvedic principles in your daily routine, emphasizing the importance of mindful eating, proper sleep, and rejuvenating self-care practices. We explore the therapeutic power of Ayurvedic herbs, the transformative practice of yoga, and the art of finding balance in an ever-changing world.

Nutrition takes center stage as we delve into the intricacies of Ayurvedic dietary principles. We decode the six tastes and their effects on the doshas, empowering you to make conscious food choices that nourish your body and mind. We also unlock the secrets of Ayurvedic cooking methods and spices, providing you with the tools to create delicious, healing meals in your own kitchen.

Ayurveda's wisdom extends beyond the physical realm, delving into the profound interplay between psychology and well-being. We explore the impact of emotions on health and delve into mindfulness practices and meditation techniques that promote emotional balance and mental clarity. Through the lens of Ayurveda, we unravel the beauty of the mind-body connection and guide you towards cultivating a positive mindset and deepening self-awareness.

Recognizing the unique needs of women's health, we dedicate a chapter to Ayurvedic approaches for menstrual health, hormonal balance, and various stages of a woman's life. We also explore the role of Ayurveda in relationships, nurturing harmonious connections and cultivating compassionate communication within our families, partnerships, and communities.

As we navigate the demands of the modern world, we explore ways to integrate Ayurveda into our fast-paced lifestyles while maintaining balance and harmony. We shed light on Ayurvedic perspectives on chronic diseases, technology, and environmental sustainability, empowering you to create a life that is aligned with your deepest values and aspirations.

Throughout this book, we provide practical tips, self-assessment tools, and nourishing recipes to support you on your Ayurvedic journey. However, it is important to remember that Ayurveda is a holistic system and should not replace professional medical advice. We encourage you to consult a qualified Ayurvedic practitioner or healthcare provider before making any significant changes to your health routine.

Are you ready to embark on a transformative path towards vibrant living and inner harmony? Let us delve into the timeless wisdom of Ayurveda, allowing its profound teachings to illuminate our lives and awaken the healer within. Together, let us unlock the gates to radiant well-being and embrace a life filled with balance, purpose, and joy.

Outline of the Book

Chapter 1: Introduction:

- The journey to wellness
- Ayurveda as a holistic approach
- Overview of the book's contents

Chapter 2: The Essence of Ayurveda

- Understanding Ayurveda's Origin and Philosophy
- The interconnectedness of mind, body, and spirit
- The five elements and the doshas: Vata, Pitta, and Kapha

- Recognizing your unique constitution (Prakriti)
- The concept of balance (Prakriti) and imbalance (Vikruti)

Chapter 3: Ayurvedic Lifestyle Principles

- The daily routine (Dinacharya) for optimal health
- The significance of proper sleep and rest
- Mindful eating and the importance of digestion (Agni)
- Ayurvedic herbs and their healing properties
- The role of exercise and movement (Yoga)

Chapter 4: Ayurvedic Nutrition

- The art of mindful eating and conscious food choices
- The six tastes and their effects on the doshas
- Designing a balanced Ayurvedic diet for your constitution
- Ayurvedic cooking methods and spices for therapeutic benefits
- Ayurvedic approaches to fasting and detoxification

Chapter 5: Ayurvedic Psychology

- Understanding the mind-body connection
- The impact of emotions and mental states on health
- Ayurvedic practices for stress reduction and relaxation
- Meditation and mindfulness techniques for emotional well-being
- Developing a positive mindset and cultivating self-awareness

Chapter 6: Ayurvedic Beauty and Self-Care

- Nurturing the body through Ayurvedic self-care rituals (Abhyanga, Neti, etc.)
- Ayurvedic skincare and natural beauty remedies
- Hair and scalp care using Ayurvedic principles
- Ayurvedic practices for maintaining oral health
- Ayurvedic approaches to aging gracefully

Chapter 7: Ayurveda for Women's Health

- Understanding the unique needs of women's health
- Ayurvedic practices for menstrual health and hormonal balance
- Preconception and pregnancy care in Ayurveda
- Postpartum rejuvenation and self-care practices
- Ayurvedic support for menopause and healthy aging in women

Chapter 8: Ayurveda and Relationships

- The Ayurvedic perspective on relationships
- Nurturing healthy communication and emotional intimacy
- Ayurvedic practices for maintaining harmony in partnerships
- Applying Ayurveda in family and community settings
- Enhancing compassion and connection through Ayurveda

Chapter 9: Ayurveda for the Modern World

- Integrating Ayurveda into a fast-paced lifestyle
- Ayurveda and technology: finding balance in a digital age
- Ayurvedic approaches to managing chronic diseases
- Ayurvedic perspectives on environmental sustainability
- Cultivating a harmonious and purposeful life

Conclusion:

- Embracing Ayurveda as a lifelong journey
- The transformative power of Ayurveda in everyday life
- Practical tips for incorporating Ayurvedic wisdom

Appendix:

- Resources for further exploration and study
- Glossary of Ayurvedic terms
- Sample Ayurvedic recipes and meal plans
- Ayurvedic self-assessment tools and quizzes

Disclaimer: The information in this book is intended for educational purposes only and should not replace professional medical advice. Consult a qualified Ayurvedic practitioner or healthcare provider before making any changes to your health routine.

CHAPTER TWO

The Essence of Ayurveda

- Understanding Ayurveda's Origin and Philosophy
- The interconnectedness of mind, body, and spirit
- The five elements and the doshas: Vata, Pitta, and Kapha
- Recognizing your unique constitution (Prakriti)
- The concept of balance (Prakriti) and imbalance (Vikruti)

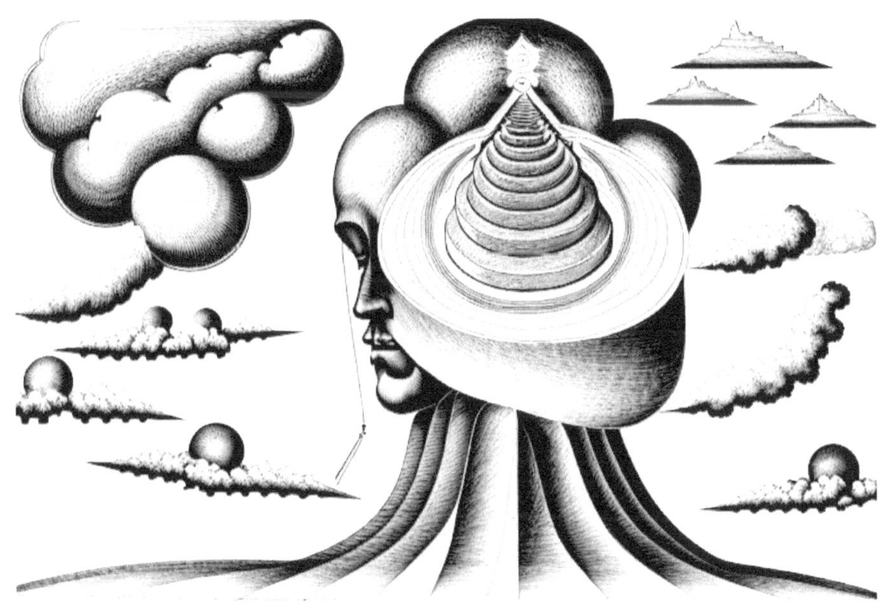

Descent of Knowledge

Understanding Ayurveda's Origin and Philosophy: Unlocking the Secrets of Holistic Well-being

The Story and the Science Behind!

According to ancient Hindu scriptures and traditions, Ayurveda, the traditional system of medicine in India, is believed to have descended from the divine realm to humans through a series of transmissions. The lineage of Ayurvedic knowledge can be traced back to the creator of the universe, Brahma, and follows a path that encompasses several key figures and divine beings.

As the story goes, Brahma, the supreme deity in Hinduism, is said to have first revealed the knowledge of Ayurveda to Daksha Prajapati, one of the ten Prajapatis or progenitors of the human race. Daksha, in turn, passed this knowledge down to the Ashwini Kumaras, who were divine physicians and the twin sons of Surya, the Sun God.

The Ashwini Kumaras, known for their exceptional healing abilities and expertise in medicine, then further disseminated the wisdom of Ayurveda to Indra, the king of the gods in Hindu mythology. Indra, being the ruler of the celestial realm, received this profound knowledge and became well-versed in the principles and practices of Ayurveda.

From Indra, the lineage of Ayurveda passed on to the sage Bharadwaja. It is said that when human beings started experiencing various health issues due to the urban lifestyle and modern living, a gathering of sages took place in the Himalayas. Among those sages was Bharadwaja, who received the sacred teachings of Ayurveda from Indra himself. Bharadwaja diligently absorbed and preserved this divine knowledge, becoming one of the foremost authorities on Ayurvedic medicine.

The transmission of Ayurveda from Brahma to Daksha, the Ashwini Kumaras, Indra, and ultimately to Bharadwaja, symbolizes the lineage of this ancient healing system. It suggests a sacred connection between the divine realm and human existence and a continuous passing down of wisdom through generations.

In addition to this historical lineage, Ayurveda also emphasizes the importance of individual spiritual growth and self-awareness. According to Ayurvedic philosophy, when we raise our consciousness to higher levels through practices such as meditation, self-reflection, and self-discipline, we become more receptive to receiving knowledge and insights from higher realms.

By expanding our consciousness and raising our vibrational frequency, we open ourselves up to a deeper understanding of the world and its interconnectedness. In this elevated state of awareness, we can access profound wisdom and insights that can guide us in various aspects of life, including health and well-being.

Therefore, in the context of Ayurveda, the ascent of knowledge to higher levels of consciousness signifies the potential for individuals to tap into universal truths and ancient wisdom, which can positively impact their physical, mental, and spiritual well-being.

It is important to note that while Ayurveda has a rich and storied history, its efficacy and relevance have been evaluated through modern scientific research and clinical studies. Today, Ayurvedic principles are widely practiced and integrated with contemporary medicine to promote holistic health and well-being.

In conclusion, Ayurveda is believed to have descended from Brahma to Daksha, then to the Ashwini Kumaras, and further to Indra before reaching the sage Bharadwaja. This lineage represents the transmission of Ayurvedic knowledge from the divine realm to humanity. Additionally, raising our consciousness to higher levels can enhance our receptivity to wisdom and insights, enabling us to access profound knowledge and lead more balanced and fulfilling lives.

Thus, in the pursuit of optimal well-being, there are ancient systems of healing that offer timeless wisdom and guidance. Among these, Ayurveda stands out as a beacon of hope, providing a comprehensive approach to balance and harmony. Rooted in the ancient scriptures of India, Ayurveda has endured for thousands of years, guiding individuals towards vibrant health and vitality. In this article, we will delve into the origin and philosophy of Ayurveda, unraveling its profound principles to empower you in your daily life.

Ayurveda, derived from the Sanskrit language, can be understood as the "science of life." The word "Ayur" translates to life, while "Veda" refers to knowledge or science. Ayurveda encompasses both the physical and metaphysical aspects of life, offering a holistic perspective on well-being.

To truly grasp the depth of Ayurveda, we must explore its historical origins. The ancient texts known as the Vedas, particularly the Rigveda and Atharvaveda, provide glimpses into the principles and practices of

Ayurveda. The sages or Rishis are credited with channeling this knowledge from the cosmos and documenting it for the benefit of humanity.

At the core of Ayurveda lie the principles of the Panchamahabhutas, the five fundamental elements: space (akasha), air (vayu), fire (tejas), water (jala), and earth (prithvi). These elements combine in various proportions to form the three doshas: Vata, Pitta, and Kapha. Each individual possesses a unique constitution, influenced by these doshas, which manifest differently in each person. Understanding your dominant dosha can help tailor lifestyle choices for optimal well-being.

Agni, the digestive fire, plays a vital role in Ayurveda. It governs digestion, assimilation, and transformation at both physical and emotional levels. A balanced agni supports vibrant health, while imbalances can lead to various ailments. Nurturing agni through mindful eating, appropriate food combinations, and digestion-enhancing herbs can promote optimal well-being.

Ayurveda emphasizes the importance of harmonizing daily routines with the natural rhythms of the day through practices known as Dinacharya. Waking up early, tongue scraping, oil pulling, self-massage (abhyanga), and mindful bathing are recommended rituals that can enhance vitality and cultivate a deeper connection with the body and mind.

Ritucharya, another aspect of Ayurveda, encourages aligning our lifestyle and dietary habits with the changing seasons. By embracing season-specific practices, we can adapt to the climate's demands and nurture our inner equilibrium.

Ayurveda views food as medicine, highlighting the importance of mindful eating for optimal health. Ahara, the Ayurvedic approach to nutrition, guides us in choosing wholesome, seasonal, and balanced meals while considering our unique constitution. It emphasizes the six tastes (rasas) and their influence on our doshas, fostering a holistic approach to nourishment.

The healing potential of Ayurveda extends beyond nutrition. Herbal medicine, using the potent properties of herbs and botanicals, is widely employed to restore balance and vitality. Ashwagandha, Turmeric, Triphala, Brahmi, and Tulsi are just a few examples of herbs with therapeutic properties.

Ayurveda and Yoga share common origins and intertwine seamlessly. Yoga, through asanas (postures), pranayama (breathing exercises), and meditation, harmonizes the body, mind, and spirit. These practices can align with your unique constitution to promote physical strength, mental clarity, and spiritual growth.

Ayurvedic body therapies, such as Panchakarma, Abhyanga (self-massage), Shirodhara (oil pouring on the forehead), and Swedana (herbal steam therapy), offer profound healing experiences. These therapies detoxify, rejuvenate, and balance the body, mind, and spirit, promoting deep relaxation and restoration.

Ayurveda recognizes the intricate interplay between our mental and physical well-being. It offers perspectives on emotions and provides tools to nurture emotional balance through self-awareness, stress management, and the cultivation of positive emotions.

Rasayana, the science of rejuvenation, focuses on preserving youthfulness and promoting longevity. Ayurvedic rejuvenation therapies incorporate practices and herbs that support vibrant health and the unfolding of one's true potential.

In conclusion, Ayurveda's origin and philosophy provide a roadmap to holistic well-being that encompasses every aspect of our lives. By embracing the wisdom of Ayurveda, we can create a harmonious existence, aligning with the rhythms of nature and nurturing our innate healing potential. Let Ayurveda be your guide on the journey towards vibrant health, balance, and inner transformation.

The Interconnectedness of Mind, Body, and Spirit: Embracing Wholeness for Holistic Well-being

In our busy lives, we often forget the profound interconnectedness of our mind, body, and spirit. We get caught up in the demands of the external world, neglecting the deeper dimensions of our being. Yet, when we awaken to the unity of these three aspects of ourselves, we unlock the gateway to true holistic well-being. It is through understanding and nurturing this interconnectedness that we can experience profound transformation and live a more fulfilling and vibrant existence.

The mind, body, and spirit are not separate entities; they are deeply intertwined and inseparable. The mind encompasses our thoughts, emotions, beliefs, and consciousness. It is the realm of our intellect, perceptions, and the seat of our awareness. The body is our physical form, the tangible vessel through which we experience the world. It houses our organs, senses, and nervous system, enabling us to engage with the physical realm. The spirit, often referred to as the soul or essence of our being, is the eternal, transcendent aspect that connects us to the divine and the infinite.

Understanding the unity of mind, body, and spirit is a fundamental step towards embracing holistic well-being. When we recognize that these aspects are intricately intertwined, we can no longer view ourselves as fragmented beings but as integrated wholes. Our thoughts and emotions affect our physical health, and our physical well-being can profoundly impact our state of mind and spiritual connection. Recognizing this interconnectedness empowers us to take a more holistic approach to our health and happiness.

Science has also begun to validate the mind-body-spirit connection, shedding light on the tangible impact of our thoughts, emotions, and beliefs on our physiology. The field of psychoneuroimmunology, for instance, explores the relationship between our mental and emotional states and our immune system, hormones, and overall health. Studies have shown that stress, negative emotions, and limiting beliefs can weaken our immune system and contribute to the onset of illness. Conversely, positive emotions, a healthy mindset, and spiritual practices have been found to enhance our well-being and support our physical health. These scientific findings provide further evidence of the undeniable influence of the mind-body-spirit connection on our overall well-being.

So, how can we embrace this interconnectedness and integrate it into our daily lives? Here are some practical insights and practices to help you embark on this transformative journey:

1. Cultivate Mindfulness: Develop a regular mindfulness practice to become more aware of your thoughts, emotions, and physical sensations. Mindfulness allows you to observe the interplay between your mind, body, and spirit without judgment, fostering a deeper understanding of your inner landscape.

2. Nourish Your Body: Pay attention to what you eat and how it affects your physical and mental well-being. Choose whole, nutrient-rich foods that nourish your body and support its natural balance. Engage in regular physical activity to keep your body vibrant and energized.

3. Embrace Emotional Intelligence: Cultivate emotional intelligence by developing an awareness of your emotions, their triggers, and their impact on your well-being. Practice self-care, engage in activities that bring you joy,

and develop healthy coping mechanisms to navigate challenging emotions.

4. Engage in Spiritual Practices: Explore spiritual practices that resonate with you, such as meditation, prayer, or connecting with nature. These practices provide a gateway to tap into the deeper dimensions of your being, fostering a sense of purpose, peace, and connection.

5. Foster Positive Relationships: Surround yourself with positive and supportive relationships. Engage in meaningful connections that uplift your spirit and contribute to your overall well-being. Nurture compassion, empathy, and love in your interactions with others.

6. Prioritize Self-Care: Take time for self-care and self-reflection. Engage in activities that promote relaxation, rejuvenation, and self-discovery. Prioritize restful sleep, practice self-compassion, and engage in activities that replenish your energy.

7. Seek Balance: Strive for balance in all aspects of your life. Attend to your physical, mental, and spiritual needs with equal care. Find harmony between work and play, solitude and social interaction, and activity and rest.

By embracing the interconnectedness of mind, body, and spirit, we unlock the potential for profound transformation and holistic well-being. As we integrate this awareness into our daily lives, we embark on a journey of self-discovery, self-healing, and self-realization. We become active participants in our own well-being, nurturing the unity of mind, body, and spirit to live a more fulfilling and vibrant existence.

The Five Elements and the Doshas: Exploring Vata, Pitta, and Kapha for Balance and Well-being

In the ancient healing system of Ayurveda, the five elements and the doshas play a central role in understanding our unique constitution and maintaining optimal health. The five elements - space, air, fire, water, and earth - are fundamental building blocks of creation, and they manifest in different combinations within each individual. These combinations give rise to the three doshas: Vata, Pitta, and Kapha. Understanding these doshas and their interplay is key to achieving balance, harmony, and well-being. In this article, we explore the five elements and delve into the characteristics of Vata, Pitta, and Kapha, offering insights on how to nurture and balance these energies in our lives.

The Five Elements: Space, Air, Fire, Water, and Earth

According to Ayurveda, the five elements form the basis of all matter, including our bodies and the natural world. Each element possesses unique qualities that contribute to our physical and energetic makeup:

1. Space (Akasha): Space represents the infinite, boundless potential that exists within and around us. It provides the container for all other elements and is associated with openness, expansion, and clarity.

2. Air (Vayu): Air is characterized by movement, lightness, and changeability. It governs activities such as breathing, circulation, and communication. Air is dynamic, adaptable, and associated with creativity and quick thinking.

3. Fire (Tejas): Fire represents transformation, heat, and energy. It provides the power of digestion, metabolism, and transformation in both the physical and mental realms. Fire is associated with passion, intensity, and the spark of inspiration.

4. Water (Jala): Water embodies fluidity, cohesion, and nourishment. It provides the vital essence for all bodily functions, including hydration, lubrication, and transportation. Water is associated with emotions, adaptability, and the flow of energy.

5. Earth (Prithvi): Earth represents stability, solidity, and groundedness. It forms the structure and foundation of our bodies and provides a sense of rootedness, strength, and nourishment. Earth is associated with material abundance, endurance, and practicality.

Understanding the Doshas: Vata, Pitta, and Kapha

The doshas are energetic forces that are derived from the combinations of the five elements. They are present in varying degrees within each individual, influencing our physical, mental, and emotional traits. The three primary doshas are Vata, Pitta, and Kapha. Let's explore the characteristics of each dosha:

1. Vata:

Vata is predominantly composed of space and air elements. It governs movement, creativity, and the nervous system. Individuals with a Vata constitution tend to be enthusiastic, creative, and quick-thinking. They often have a slender build, dry skin, and a tendency towards coldness. When in balance, Vata types are vibrant, flexible, and full of energy. However, when imbalanced, they may experience anxiety, restlessness, digestive issues, and insomnia.

To balance Vata, it is important to prioritize grounding practices, establish a regular routine, eat warm and nourishing foods, and engage in calming activities such as gentle yoga, meditation, and self-care rituals.

2. Pitta:

Pitta is primarily composed of fire and water elements. It governs digestion, metabolism, and transformation. Pitta types are often characterized by their intensity, focus, and strong drive. They tend to have a medium build, warm body temperature, and a radiant complexion. When in balance, Pitta types are intelligent, goal-oriented, and have a strong digestion. However, when imbalanced, they may experience irritability, anger, inflammation, and digestive disturbances.

To balance Pitta, it is important to adopt cooling practices, maintain a balanced schedule, eat cooling and hydrating foods, and engage in activities that promote relaxation and moderation, such as swimming, spending time in nature, and practicing mindfulness.

3. Kapha:

Kapha is primarily composed of water and earth elements. It governs stability, structure, and lubrication in the body. Kapha types are often characterized by their calmness, strength, and nurturing nature. They tend to have a solid build, soft skin, and a steady energy. When in balance, Kapha types are compassionate, grounded, and have excellent stamina. However, when imbalanced, they may experience lethargy, weight gain, congestion, and attachment.

To balance Kapha, it is important to embrace invigorating practices, engage in regular exercise, eat light and warming foods, and cultivate mental and physical stimulation through activities such as dancing, hiking, and trying new experiences.

Understanding our unique doshic constitution is key to making lifestyle choices that support our individual needs. While we each have a dominant dosha, it's common to have a combination of two or even all three doshas. The goal is to achieve harmony and balance among the doshas, which will vary for each person.

In Conclusion:

The five elements and the doshas are essential components of Ayurvedic philosophy, providing us with a framework for understanding our individual nature and promoting holistic well-being. By recognizing the qualities and characteristics of Vata, Pitta, and Kapha, we can make informed choices about diet, lifestyle, and self-care practices to create balance and harmony in our lives. Embracing this knowledge allows us to nurture our mind, body, and spirit, leading to a greater sense of vitality, peace, and overall well-being.

Recognizing Your Unique Constitution (Prakriti): Embracing Ayurveda's Path to Optimal Health and Well-being

In the ancient healing system of Ayurveda, recognizing and understanding your unique constitution, known as Prakriti, is a foundational step towards achieving optimal health and well-being. Prakriti refers to your inherent physical, mental, and energetic makeup—the blueprint that governs your unique strengths, vulnerabilities, and tendencies. By recognizing and honoring your Prakriti, you can make informed choices about diet, lifestyle, and self-care practices that support your individual needs. In this article, we explore the significance of Prakriti and offer insights on how to recognize and embrace your unique constitution for a balanced and fulfilling life.

The Essence of Prakriti: Understanding Your Blueprint

Prakriti encompasses the fundamental aspects of your being, including physical attributes, temperament, emotional tendencies, and energy patterns. It is determined by the combination of the three doshas—Vata, Pitta, and Kapha—that are present within you from birth. Each dosha is associated with specific elements and qualities, and the unique blend of these doshas forms your Prakriti.

Recognizing Your Prakriti: A Journey of Self-Discovery

Discovering your Prakriti is a journey of self-discovery that involves observing and understanding your physical, mental, and emotional traits. Here are some key aspects to consider when recognizing your Prakriti:

1. Physical Characteristics: Observe your body structure, body weight, metabolism, and natural inclinations. Are you naturally slender or more solidly built? Do you tend to gain or lose weight easily? Are your skin, hair, and nails dry or oily? These observations can provide clues about your dominant dosha(s).

2. Temperament and Personality: Pay attention to your innate temperament and emotional tendencies. Are you naturally calm and grounded, or do you have a fiery and passionate nature? Are you prone to worry and anxiety, or are you more easygoing and adaptable? Understanding these traits can help you identify the dosha(s) that are most prevalent within you.

3. Energy Patterns: Notice your energy levels throughout the day. Do you have bursts of energy followed by periods of fatigue? Are you naturally

active and restless, or do you have a steady and consistent energy flow? These energy patterns can provide insights into your doshic constitution.

4. Response to Stress: Observe how you respond to stressors in your life. Do you become anxious and overwhelmed (Vata response), or do you become irritable and easily angered (Pitta response)? Alternatively, do you tend to withdraw and become emotionally stagnant (Kapha response)? Recognizing your stress response can shed light on your dominant dosha(s).

Consulting an Ayurvedic Practitioner: Seeking Guidance
While self-observation is valuable, consulting an experienced Ayurvedic practitioner can provide further clarity and guidance in recognizing your Prakriti. An Ayurvedic practitioner will use diagnostic tools, such as pulse diagnosis, questionnaires, and detailed consultations, to assess your doshic balance and determine your unique constitution.

Embracing Your Prakriti: Nurturing Balance and Well-being
Once you have recognized your Prakriti, the next step is to embrace it and make lifestyle choices that support your unique constitution. Here are some practical tips for nurturing balance and well-being based on your dominant dosha(s):

1. Vata:
- Create a regular routine and stick to it.
- Prioritize grounding practices, such as yoga, tai chi, or walking in nature.
- Eat warm, nourishing foods and avoid raw or cold foods.
- Engage in calming activities, like meditation and gentle self-massage.

2. Pitta:
- Maintain a balanced schedule with time for relaxation and leisure.
- Incorporate cooling practices, such as swimming or spending time in nature.
- Opt for cooling, hydrating foods and minimize spicy or oily foods.
- Cultivate mindfulness and engage in activities that promote emotional balance.

3. Kapha:
- Stay physically active with regular exercise and movement.
- Choose light, warm, and spicy foods and minimize heavy or oily foods.
- Stimulate your mind and body with mental and physical challenges.
- Embrace variety and change in your routines and activities.

Remember, the goal is to achieve balance and harmony among the doshas, and the specific recommendations may vary depending on your unique Prakriti. Regular self-reflection and adaptation to changing circumstances are essential to maintain equilibrium.

In Conclusion: Embrace Your Prakriti, Embrace Your Wholeness
Recognizing your unique constitution, or Prakriti, is a powerful step towards achieving optimal health and well-being. By understanding the characteristics and tendencies associated with your dominant dosha(s), you can make informed choices that support your individual needs. Embrace your Prakriti as a roadmap to self-discovery and self-care, and cultivate a harmonious balance among the doshas. As you align with your true nature, you unlock the potential for vitality, inner peace, and holistic well-being.

The Concept of Balance (Prakriti) and Imbalance (Vikruti): Restoring Harmony in Ayurveda

In the ancient healing tradition of Ayurveda, the concept of balance (Prakriti) and imbalance (Vikruti) forms the cornerstone of holistic health and well-being. Ayurveda recognizes that maintaining a state of equilibrium within our body, mind, and spirit is essential for optimal health, while imbalances can lead to disharmony and disease. In this article, we delve into the concepts of Prakriti and Vikruti, exploring their significance and offering insights on how to restore balance and promote overall well-being.

Prakriti: The State of Natural Balance
Prakriti refers to our inherent, natural state of balance. It is our unique constitution—the combination of physical, mental, and energetic characteristics that we are born with. Prakriti is determined by the predominance of the three doshas—Vata, Pitta, and Kapha—in our individual makeup. When our doshas are in balance, we experience a sense of well-being, vitality, and harmony. Our body functions optimally, our mind is clear and focused, and our energy flows smoothly.

Recognizing and understanding our Prakriti is crucial because it guides us in making choices that support our individual needs for diet, lifestyle, and self-care practices. It empowers us to live in alignment with our true nature and maintain overall health and vitality.

Vikruti: The State of Imbalance
While Prakriti represents our natural state of balance, Vikruti refers to the state of imbalance or disharmony that occurs when our doshas become disturbed. Vikruti can be influenced by various factors, including diet, lifestyle, emotional state, environmental conditions, and external stressors.

When our doshas are imbalanced, we may experience a range of physical, mental, and emotional symptoms that indicate a state of Vikruti.

Recognizing Vikruti is essential for understanding the root cause of any health issues or imbalances we may be facing. It helps us identify the doshas that are out of balance and provides insights into the areas of our life that require attention and adjustment.

Restoring Balance: The Path to Well-being

The goal of Ayurveda is to restore balance and harmony within the body, mind, and spirit. When we address the imbalances indicated by Vikruti, we can bring ourselves back to a state of Prakriti, where optimal health and well-being reside. Here are some key principles and practices to restore balance:

1. Self-Reflection and Awareness: Cultivate self-awareness by regularly observing and reflecting on your physical, mental, and emotional states. Notice any signs of imbalance, such as digestive issues, sleep disturbances, stress, or emotional fluctuations. This awareness is the first step toward restoring balance.

2. Ayurvedic Lifestyle and Diet: Embrace an Ayurvedic lifestyle that supports your unique Prakriti and addresses your imbalances. Follow a diet that is appropriate for your doshic constitution and incorporate daily self-care practices, such as oil massage, tongue scraping, and meditation. Establishing a regular routine and engaging in activities that promote relaxation and rejuvenation are also vital.

3. Herbal Support: Ayurveda offers a wealth of herbs and herbal formulations that can help restore balance to the doshas. Consult with an experienced Ayurvedic practitioner to determine the specific herbs or herbal remedies that are appropriate for your Vikruti and support your journey toward balance.

4. Mind-Body Practices: Engage in mind-body practices that promote balance and well-being, such as yoga, pranayama (breathing exercises), and meditation. These practices help calm the mind, reduce stress, and balance the doshas, bringing about a sense of inner harmony.

5. Seek Professional Guidance: Working with an experienced Ayurvedic practitioner can provide valuable insights and guidance tailored to your unique needs. They can help assess your Prakriti and Vikruti, offer personalized recommendations, and monitor your progress on the path to restoring balance.

Remember, balance is not a static state but a dynamic process. It requires constant self-awareness, adaptation, and conscious choices. Each individual's journey toward balance is unique, and it may take time and patience to restore equilibrium. Embrace the process as an opportunity for self-discovery and transformation, and celebrate the small steps you take towards creating a harmonious and healthy life.

In Conclusion: Nurturing Balance, Cultivating Well-being

The concepts of Prakriti and Vikruti in Ayurveda emphasize the importance of maintaining balance within our body, mind, and spirit. By recognizing and addressing imbalances indicated by Vikruti, we can restore harmony and promote overall well-being. Embrace Ayurvedic principles, lifestyle practices, and self-care rituals to support your unique Prakriti and bring yourself back to a state of balance. Embody the wisdom of Ayurveda, nurture your innate equilibrium, and embark on a transformative journey towards optimal health and holistic well-being.

CHAPTER THREE

Ayurvedic Lifestyle Principles

- The daily routine (Dinacharya) for optimal health
- The significance of proper sleep and rest
- Mindful eating and the importance of digestion (Agni)
- Ayurvedic herbs and their healing properties
- The role of Vyayama, exercise and movement (Yogasana)

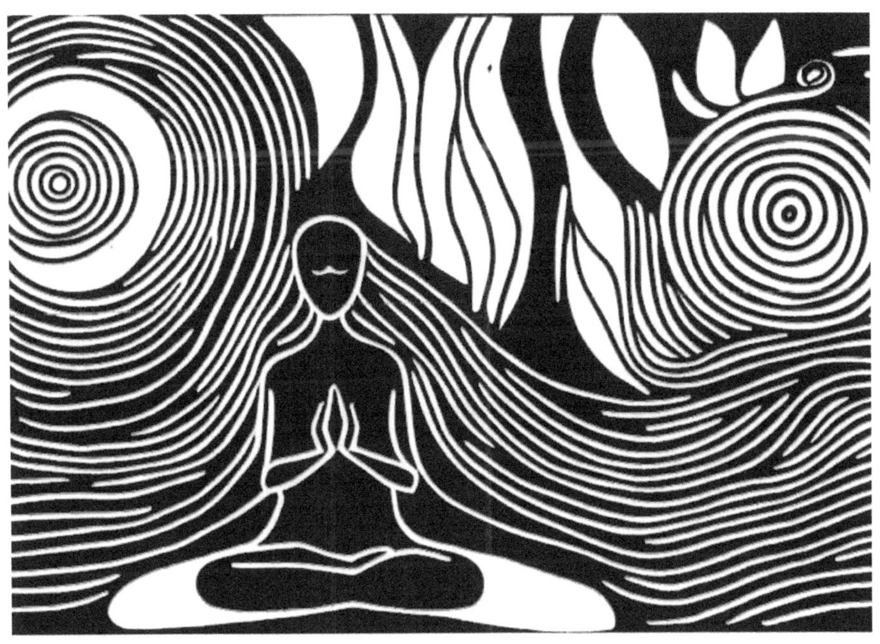

Body, Mind & Soul

In the ancient healing system of Ayurveda, optimal health and well-being are achieved through the harmonious integration of body, mind, and spirit. Ayurveda recognizes the interconnectedness of all aspects of our being and provides us with a comprehensive framework to cultivate balance and vitality in our daily lives. At the core of Ayurvedic lifestyle principles lie the concepts of the daily routine (Dinacharya), restful sleep, mindful eating and digestion (Agni), the healing properties of Ayurvedic herbs, and the role of exercise and movement, particularly through the practice of Yoga. In this article, we explore these essential elements and their significance in promoting optimal health.

Incorporating Ayurvedic lifestyle principles into our daily lives empowers us to take an active role in nurturing our health and well-being. By embracing a daily routine that supports our natural rhythms, prioritizing restful sleep, practicing mindful eating and digestion, harnessing the healing properties of Ayurvedic herbs, and engaging in regular exercise and movement, we can cultivate a state of balance and vitality. Ayurveda offers us a comprehensive and holistic approach to optimal health, allowing us to thrive in all aspects of our lives.

The Daily Routine (Dinacharya) for Optimal Health: Embracing Ayurvedic Lifestyle Principles

In our fast-paced and hectic lives, finding balance and maintaining optimal health can often feel like a challenge. However, the ancient healing system of Ayurveda offers a powerful solution in the form of a daily routine known as Dinacharya. Rooted in the principles of Ayurveda, Dinacharya provides a comprehensive framework for promoting physical, mental, and spiritual well-being through simple yet profound practices. In this article, we explore the significance of Dinacharya and how you can incorporate it into your life to cultivate optimal health.

What is Dinacharya?

Dinacharya refers to a set of daily practices and routines that are aligned with the natural rhythms of the day. It is believed that following a consistent and mindful daily routine helps to balance the doshas (Vata, Pitta, and Kapha), improve digestion, enhance energy levels, boost immunity, promote mental clarity, and establish a sense of grounding and stability.

The Morning Routine:

The way we start our day sets the tone for the rest of it. Ayurveda places great importance on establishing a morning routine that nurtures and energizes us. Here are some key practices to incorporate into your morning routine:

1. Rise Early: Wake up before sunrise, ideally during the Vata time of day (before 6 a.m.). This allows you to align with the natural rhythm of the day and experience the calm and stillness of the early morning.

2. Tongue Scraping: Upon waking, gently scrape your tongue with a tongue scraper. This simple practice removes toxins that have accumulated overnight, promotes oral hygiene, and stimulates digestion.

3. Oil Pulling: Swish a tablespoon of warm sesame or coconut oil in your mouth for 5-10 minutes. This Ayurvedic technique helps to remove bacteria, improve oral health, and promote overall detoxification.

4. Hydration: Start your day by drinking a glass of warm water with lemon to hydrate your body, stimulate digestion, and support detoxification. Note that the amount of water intake depends on several factors like Prakriti, season, digestive capacity (Agni), the type of food consumed, physical activity, and so on.

5. Self-Massage (Abhyanga): Massage your body with warm oil, such as sesame or coconut oil, before showering. This practice nourishes the skin, calms the nervous system, improves circulation, and promotes overall relaxation.

6. Bathing: Take a refreshing shower or bath to cleanse your body and awaken your senses. You can use natural soaps or herbal formulations to enhance the therapeutic benefits.

7. Meditation and Mindfulness: Dedicate a few minutes to meditation, deep breathing, or mindfulness practices. This allows you to center yourself, cultivate mental clarity, and set positive intentions for the day ahead.

The Daytime Routine:
Throughout the day, it is essential to maintain a balanced and mindful approach to your activities. Here are some key practices to incorporate into your daytime routine:

1. Balanced Meals: Enjoy nourishing meals that are appropriate for your dosha type and are freshly prepared. Emphasize whole foods, seasonal fruits and vegetables, and incorporate the six tastes (sweet, sour, salty, pungent, bitter, and astringent) to ensure a balanced diet.

2. Regular Meal Times: Establish regular meal times and aim to eat your meals at a relaxed pace. Avoid distractions such as screens or work during mealtime and focus on savoring the flavors and textures of your food.

3. Stay Hydrated: Drink warm or room temperature water throughout the day to stay hydrated and support digestion. Avoid drinking excessive amounts of cold or iced beverages, as they can disrupt the digestive fire. Note that the amount of water intake depends on several factors like Prakriti, season, digestive capacity (Agni), the type of food consumed, physical activity, and so on.

4. Mindful Breaks: Take short breaks throughout the day to rest, stretch, and reset your mind. This can involve taking a walk in nature, practicing deep breathing exercises, or engaging in a few minutes of meditation or mindfulness.

5. Honor Natural Urges: Pay attention to your body's natural urges, such as urination and elimination. Respond to these urges promptly to support healthy digestion and elimination processes.

The Evening Routine:

As the day winds down, it is important to create a nurturing evening routine that promotes relaxation and prepares you for restful sleep. Here are some practices to incorporate into your evening routine:

1. Light Dinners: Opt for a light and easily digestible dinner, preferably a few hours before bedtime. This allows your body to focus on the process of digestion without being overloaded.

2. Digital Detox: Disconnect from electronic devices at least an hour before bedtime. The blue light emitted by screens can disrupt your sleep-wake cycle and interfere with your ability to unwind and prepare for sleep.

3. Relaxation Practices: Engage in activities that promote relaxation and calmness, such as reading a book, taking a warm bath, practicing gentle stretching or yoga, or enjoying a soothing cup of herbal tea.

4. Create a Sleep Sanctuary: Make your bedroom a peaceful and comfortable space that promotes restful sleep. Keep the room dark, quiet, and at a cool temperature. Consider using essential oils, such as lavender or chamomile, to create a soothing atmosphere.

5. Consistent Bedtime: Aim to go to bed at the same time each night, ideally before 10 p.m. This allows you to align with the natural rhythms of the body and experience the most restorative sleep.

Incorporating Dinacharya into your daily life may require some adjustments and a commitment to consistent practice. However, the benefits it offers in terms of physical, mental, and spiritual well-being are profound. By embracing a mindful and balanced daily routine, you can cultivate optimal health, enhance your energy levels, improve your digestion, and experience a deep sense of overall well-being.

Remember, Ayurveda recognizes that each individual is unique, so it is essential to personalize your routine according to your specific needs and doshic constitution. Consulting with an Ayurvedic practitioner can provide valuable guidance and support on your journey to optimal health through Dinacharya. Embrace the wisdom of Ayurveda, and let the daily routine become a transformative and nourishing practice that nurtures your body, mind, and spirit.

The Significance of Proper Sleep and Rest: Unlocking Health and Vitality through Ayurvedic Wisdom

In our modern, fast-paced world, sleep often takes a backseat as we juggle countless responsibilities and commitments. However, the ancient science of Ayurveda reminds us of the profound significance of proper sleep and rest in maintaining optimal health and vitality. Ayurveda recognizes that sleep is not merely a period of inactivity but a time of rejuvenation and healing for the mind, body, and spirit. In this article, we delve into the wisdom of Ayurveda and explore the profound impact of quality sleep on our overall well-being.

Understanding Sleep from an Ayurvedic Perspective:
According to Ayurveda, sleep is one of the three pillars of life, alongside proper diet and balanced lifestyle. It is considered essential for maintaining a state of equilibrium and promoting optimal health. Ayurveda views sleep as a time when the body's natural intelligence restores, repairs, and rejuvenates itself, allowing us to awaken feeling refreshed and energized.

The Doshas and Sleep:
In Ayurveda, the doshas—Vata, Pitta, and Kapha—play a significant role in our sleep patterns and quality of rest. An imbalance in any of these doshas can disrupt sleep and lead to various health issues.

1. Vata: Vata governs movement, including the nervous system. When Vata is imbalanced, it can lead to restlessness, difficulty falling asleep, and interrupted sleep throughout the night.

2. Pitta: Pitta is associated with heat and transformation in the body. An imbalance in Pitta can result in excess heat, leading to sleep disturbances, excessive dreaming, and difficulty staying asleep.

3. Kapha: Kapha represents stability, nourishment, and grounding. When Kapha is out of balance, it can manifest as excessive sleepiness, heaviness

upon waking, and a feeling of lethargy throughout the day.

The Benefits of Proper Sleep and Rest:

1. Physical Rejuvenation: During sleep, the body repairs and regenerates tissues, supports immune function, and balances hormone levels. Proper sleep helps to enhance cellular repair, improve metabolism, and boost overall vitality.

2. Mental Clarity and Emotional Balance: Quality sleep supports cognitive function, memory consolidation, and emotional well-being. It allows the mind to process and integrate information, leading to improved focus, concentration, and emotional resilience.

3. Stress Reduction: Restful sleep plays a crucial role in managing stress and reducing anxiety. It helps to regulate stress hormones, supports the nervous system, and promotes a sense of calmness and inner peace.

4. Digestive Health: Ayurveda emphasizes the connection between sleep and digestion. Quality sleep supports healthy digestion, as it allows the body to efficiently process and eliminate waste. It also helps to balance the digestive fire (Agni), ensuring optimal nutrient absorption and preventing digestive disturbances.

Tips for Restful Sleep According to Ayurveda:

1. Establish a Consistent Sleep Schedule: Aim to go to bed and wake up at the same time each day, even on weekends. This helps to align your sleep-wake cycle with the natural rhythms of the day, promoting better sleep quality.

2. Create a Soothing Bedtime Routine: Establish a calming routine before bed to signal to your body that it is time to wind down. This may include activities such as reading, taking a warm bath, practicing gentle yoga or meditation, or enjoying a cup of herbal tea.

3. Create a Sleep-Conducive Environment: Ensure that your bedroom is dark, quiet, and at a cool temperature. Use blackout curtains, earplugs, or a white noise machine if necessary. Consider using essential oils such as lavender or chamomile to create a soothing ambiance.

4. Limit Stimulating Activities: Minimize exposure to electronic devices, intense mental stimulation, and stimulating beverages (caffeine, alcohol) in the evening. These can interfere with your ability to relax and fall asleep easily.

5. Create a Comfortable Sleep Environment: Invest in a supportive mattress, comfortable pillows, and breathable bedding. Make sure your sleep environment promotes physical relaxation and comfort.

6. Practice Relaxation Techniques: Engage in relaxation techniques such as deep breathing exercises, progressive muscle relaxation, or guided imagery before bed. These practices help to calm the nervous system and prepare the body for restful sleep.

7. Pay Attention to Diet and Lifestyle: Follow a balanced Ayurvedic diet that supports your doshic constitution and promotes healthy sleep. Avoid heavy meals, excessive caffeine or sugary foods, and late-night eating. Engage in regular exercise or movement during the day to support overall well-being and improve sleep quality.

Remember, proper sleep and rest are essential pillars of health and well-being. By honoring and prioritizing quality sleep, we nourish our bodies, rejuvenate our minds, and cultivate vitality from within. Embrace the wisdom of Ayurveda and create a nurturing sleep routine that supports your unique needs, allowing you to awaken each day with renewed energy, clarity, and a deep sense of well-being.

Mindful Eating and the Importance of Digestion (Agni): Nourishing Body, Mind, and Spirit through Ayurvedic Wisdom

In our fast-paced modern lives, eating has become a rushed and mindless activity for many of us. We often eat on the go, multitask while eating, or consume food without truly savoring its flavors and textures. However, the ancient science of Ayurveda reminds us of the profound importance of mindful eating and the role of digestion, known as Agni, in maintaining optimal health and well-being. In this article, we explore the wisdom of Ayurveda and delve into the significance of mindful eating and the digestive process.

Understanding Agni and Digestion:
In Ayurveda, Agni refers to the digestive fire that transforms food into nutrients and energy. It is considered the cornerstone of health and vitality. When Agni is balanced and strong, it efficiently digests food, eliminates waste, and supports the body's overall metabolic functions. However, when Agni is weakened or imbalanced, it can lead to digestive disturbances, nutrient deficiencies, and the accumulation of toxins in the body.

The Importance of Mindful Eating:
Mindful eating is a practice that involves paying attention to the present moment and fully engaging with the act of eating. It encourages us to slow

down, savor each bite, and develop a deeper connection with our food. Here are some reasons why mindful eating is essential for our health and well-being:

1. Improved Digestion: Mindful eating enhances the awareness of our body's signals of hunger and fullness, allowing us to eat in moderation. By chewing our food thoroughly and being present with each bite, we support the digestive process and optimize nutrient absorption.

2. Enhanced Satiety: When we eat mindfully, we become more attuned to our body's satiety cues. This helps us recognize when we are genuinely hungry and when we have had enough, preventing overeating and promoting a healthy body weight.

3. Connection with Food: Mindful eating invites us to appreciate the nourishment that food provides. It allows us to connect with the source of our food, the flavors, and the textures, fostering a sense of gratitude and reverence for the sustenance it offers.

4. Improved Relationship with Food: Mindful eating helps us develop a healthier and more balanced relationship with food. By being present and non-judgmental during meals, we can reduce emotional eating, cravings, and mindless snacking.

Tips for Practicing Mindful Eating:

1. Create a Sacred Eating Space: Designate a peaceful and clutter-free space for your meals. Set the table with care, using beautiful dishes and utensils, and create an environment that promotes relaxation and enjoyment.

2. Eat without Distractions: Minimize distractions such as screens, work, or reading while eating. Instead, focus on the sensory experience of the food, the flavors, the aromas, and the textures.

3. Chew Thoroughly: Take the time to chew your food slowly and thoroughly. Chewing breaks down the food and aids digestion, allowing the digestive enzymes in your saliva to begin their work.

4. Engage Your Senses: Before taking your first bite, take a moment to observe the colors, shapes, and textures of the food. Notice the aroma and appreciate the flavors as you savor each bite.

5. Practice Gratitude: Express gratitude for the food you are about to eat. Reflect on the efforts of those involved in producing and preparing the meal, and the nourishment it will provide your body.

6. Listen to Your Body: Pay attention to your body's signals of hunger and fullness. Eat when you are genuinely hungry and pause when you are satisfied, even if there is still food left on your plate.

The Role of Agni and Digestive Health:

Ayurveda emphasizes the importance of maintaining a balanced and strong Agni to support optimal digestion and overall health. Here are some Ayurvedic tips to promote healthy digestion:

1. Eat According to Your Dosha: Ayurveda recognizes that each person has a unique doshic constitution. Understanding your dosha can help you choose the right foods and eating habits that support your digestive balance.

2. Favor Warm, Cooked Foods: Warm, cooked foods are easier to digest and provide nourishment without taxing the digestive system. Include a variety of whole grains, vegetables, legumes, and healthy fats in your diet.

3. Spice It Up: Incorporate Ayurvedic spices such as ginger, cumin, coriander, and turmeric into your meals. These spices help to kindle Agni and aid in digestion.

4. Avoid Overeating: Respect your body's capacity and avoid overeating, which can overwhelm the digestive system and lead to digestive discomfort. Aim to eat until you are about three-quarters full to allow room for proper digestion.

5. Supportive Eating Times: Ayurveda recommends having your main meal at lunchtime when Agni is strongest. In the evening, opt for a lighter meal that is easy to digest to support restful sleep.

6. Stay Hydrated: Sip warm water throughout the day to support hydration and digestion. Avoid ice-cold beverages, as they can dampen Agni and hinder the digestive process.

7. Practice Ayurvedic Herbs: Incorporate Ayurvedic herbs such as Triphala, ginger, or fennel into your routine to support healthy digestion. Consult with an Ayurvedic practitioner to determine the best herbs for your specific needs.

By embracing mindful eating and nurturing a balanced Agni, we can experience the profound benefits of optimal digestion and overall well-being. Cultivate a deeper connection with your food, savor each bite, and honor the wisdom of Ayurveda in promoting a harmonious relationship with your body, mind, and spirit. Remember, the act of eating is not only about nourishing the physical body but also nourishing the soul.

Ayurvedic Herbs and Their Healing Properties: Harnessing Nature's Wisdom for Optimal Health and Well-being

For thousands of years, Ayurveda, the ancient Indian system of medicine, has relied on the power of herbs to promote health, balance, and vitality. Ayurvedic herbs are natural remedies derived from plants, roots, leaves, and seeds, each possessing unique healing properties. These herbs are known to restore balance, support the body's natural healing processes, and promote overall well-being. In this article, we explore the wisdom of Ayurvedic herbs and their profound healing properties.

1. Ashwagandha (Withania somnifera):
Ashwagandha is considered one of the most important Ayurvedic herbs. Known as an adaptogen, it helps the body adapt to stress and promotes a sense of calmness and balance. Ashwagandha is also known to support healthy immune function, enhance vitality, and promote restful sleep.

2. Tulsi (Ocimum sanctum):
Also known as Holy Basil, Tulsi is revered in Ayurveda for its spiritual and medicinal properties. Tulsi has potent antioxidant and anti-inflammatory properties, supporting a healthy immune system and promoting respiratory health. It is also known to reduce stress, support mental clarity, and uplift the spirit.

3. Triphala:
Triphala is a combination of three fruits: Amalaki (Indian Gooseberry), Bibhitaki (Terminalia bellirica), and Haritaki (Terminalia chebula). This powerful herbal blend supports healthy digestion, detoxification, and elimination. Triphala is also known to rejuvenate the body, support healthy weight management, and promote overall vitality.

4. Turmeric (Curcuma longa):
Turmeric is a vibrant yellow spice commonly used in Ayurvedic medicine. It contains a compound called curcumin, which has potent anti-inflammatory and antioxidant properties. Turmeric supports joint health, promotes healthy digestion, supports liver function, and enhances immune health. It is also used externally for skincare and wound healing.

5. Brahmi (Bacopa monnieri):
Brahmi is a renowned Ayurvedic herb for its cognitive-enhancing properties. It supports memory, concentration, and overall brain health. Brahmi is also known to reduce anxiety, promote calmness, and support a balanced nervous system.

6. Amla (Emblica officinalis):
Also known as Indian Gooseberry, Amla is a rich source of vitamin C and antioxidants. It supports immune function, aids digestion, and promotes

healthy skin and hair. Amla is considered a rejuvenating herb that nourishes all the body's tissues and enhances vitality.

7. Neem (Azadirachta indica):
Neem is a powerful herb known for its antibacterial, antifungal, and blood-purifying properties. It supports healthy skin, helps balance blood sugar levels, supports a healthy immune system, and promotes oral health.

8. Shatavari (Asparagus racemosus):
Shatavari is a renowned Ayurvedic herb for women's health. It supports hormonal balance, reproductive health, and helps with menopause-related symptoms. Shatavari is also known for its rejuvenating and nourishing effects on the body.

9. Guduchi (Tinospora cordifolia):
Guduchi is a potent herb known for its immune-enhancing properties. It supports healthy immune function, helps purify the blood, and promotes healthy liver function. Guduchi is also used to support healthy digestion and reduce inflammation.

10. Haritaki (Terminalia chebula):
Haritaki is a powerful rejuvenating herb known as the "King of Medicines" in Ayurveda. It supports healthy digestion, promotes detoxification, enhances cognitive function, and supports overall vitality. Haritaki is also used in Ayurvedic formulations to balance the doshas.

When using Ayurvedic herbs, it is important to seek guidance from an experienced Ayurvedic practitioner who can recommend the appropriate herbs, dosages, and combinations based on your unique constitution and health needs.

Ayurvedic herbs offer a natural and holistic approach to health and well-being. These herbs embody the wisdom of nature and provide a gentle yet powerful means to support the body, mind, and spirit. Incorporating Ayurvedic herbs into your lifestyle can bring about transformative changes and help you achieve optimal health and vitality. Embrace the healing power of Ayurvedic herbs and unlock the potential for a balanced and harmonious life.

Vyayama and the Role of Exercise and Movement (Yogasana): Cultivating Physical and Mental Well-being through Ayurvedic Wisdom

In the ancient science of Ayurveda, the importance of exercise and movement in maintaining optimal health and well-being is deeply recognized. Ayurveda acknowledges that a sedentary lifestyle can lead to imbalances in the body and mind, while regular physical activity promotes strength, flexibility, and overall vitality. In this article, we explore the Ayurvedic perspective on exercise and movement, known as Vyayama, and the role of Yogasana (yoga postures) in supporting a harmonious and balanced life.

Understanding Vyayama:

Vyayama refers to physical exercise and movement practices that promote strength, flexibility, and energy circulation throughout the body. In Ayurveda, Vyayama is considered an integral part of daily routine (Dinacharya) for maintaining optimal health. It is believed that regular physical activity helps balance the doshas (Vata, Pitta, and Kapha), improves digestion, enhances metabolic function, and promotes mental clarity.

Benefits of Vyayama and Yogasana:

1. Physical Strength and Flexibility: Regular exercise and Yogasana practice help develop strength, flexibility, and endurance. It improves muscle tone, joint mobility, and overall physical performance.

2. Healthy Weight Management: Engaging in physical activity supports healthy weight management by boosting metabolism, burning calories, and reducing excess body fat. It helps maintain a healthy body composition and prevents weight-related imbalances.

3. Improved Digestion: Vyayama stimulates the digestive fire (Agni), enhancing digestion and nutrient absorption. It can help relieve digestive issues such as bloating, constipation, and indigestion.

4. Enhanced Energy and Vitality: Exercise and Yogasana practices increase prana (life force energy) circulation throughout the body, resulting in heightened energy levels, improved focus, and increased vitality.

5. Stress Reduction and Emotional Well-being: Physical activity and Yogasana are known to reduce stress, anxiety, and depression. They promote the release of endorphins, the body's natural mood-boosting hormones, and help cultivate a calm and balanced state of mind.

6. Improved Sleep Quality: Regular exercise supports healthy sleep patterns by reducing restlessness, promoting relaxation, and balancing the nervous system. It can help alleviate sleep disorders and improve overall sleep quality.

Incorporating Vyayama and Yogasana into Your Routine:

1. Choose Activities According to Your Dosha: Ayurveda recognizes that each person has a unique doshic constitution. Consider activities that align with your dosha and provide balance. For example, Vata types may benefit from gentle, grounding exercises, while Pitta types may enjoy moderate intensity workouts, and Kapha types may benefit from more vigorous activities.

2. Listen to Your Body: Pay attention to your body's signals and limitations. Engage in activities that feel comfortable and enjoyable. It's important to find a balance between challenging yourself and avoiding excessive strain or injury.

3. Practice Yogasana: Incorporate Yogasana practice into your routine to enhance flexibility, balance, and body-mind connection. Choose a style of yoga that resonates with you and seek guidance from a qualified yoga instructor.

4. Prioritize Consistency over Intensity: Consistency is key when it comes to reaping the benefits of exercise and movement. Aim for regularity in your routine rather than focusing solely on intensity or duration. Even short bouts of exercise can be beneficial when done consistently.

5. Find Joy in Movement: Engage in activities that bring you joy and make you feel alive. Whether it's dancing, walking in nature, practicing martial arts, or playing a sport, find forms of movement that resonate with your interests and passions.

6. Warm-Up and Cool Down: Before and after exercise, take the time to warm up and cool down. This helps prepare your body for physical activity and prevents injuries. Incorporate gentle stretching and relaxation techniques during the cool-down phase.

7. Rest and Recovery: Allow your body ample time to rest and recover. Balance physical activity with periods of relaxation and rejuvenation to avoid overexertion and burnout.

Remember, the aim of Vyayama and Yogasana is not only physical fitness but also the cultivation of a balanced and harmonious life. Embrace the wisdom of Ayurveda and incorporate exercise and movement practices into your daily routine. By doing so, you can promote optimal physical and mental well-being, enhance your connection with your body, and experience the profound benefits of a balanced and joyful life.

CHAPTER FOUR

Ayurvedic Nutrition

- The art of mindful eating and conscious food choices
- The six tastes and their effects on the doshas
- Designing a Balanced Ayurvedic Diet for your constitution
- Ayurvedic cooking methods and spices for therapeutic benefits
- Ayurvedic approaches to fasting and detoxification

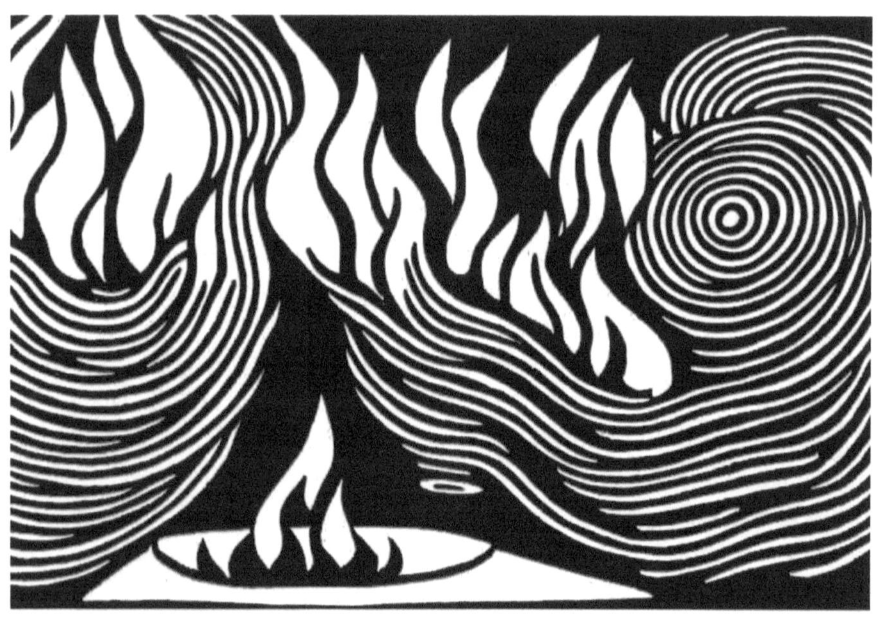

Agni (Fire) and the Fuel

In the quest for optimal health and well-being, Ayurveda offers a holistic approach that encompasses various aspects of our lives, including nutrition. Ayurvedic nutrition is a profound and ancient wisdom that recognizes the intricate relationship between food, the doshas (Vata, Pitta, and Kapha), and our overall state of well-being. It emphasizes the art of mindful eating, conscious food choices, and designing a balanced diet that supports our unique constitution. In this article, we delve into the world of Ayurvedic nutrition, exploring the six tastes, Ayurvedic cooking methods, therapeutic spices, and the role of fasting and detoxification.

Ayurvedic nutrition invites us to embark on a journey of self-discovery and self-care through conscious food choices. By embracing the principles of mindful eating, understanding the six tastes, designing a balanced diet, utilizing Ayurvedic cooking methods and spices, and incorporating fasting and detoxification practices, we can nourish our bodies and minds in a profound and transformative way. So let us embark on this Ayurvedic culinary adventure and experience the joys of vibrant health and well-being.

The Art of Mindful Eating and Conscious Food Choices: Nourishing Body and Soul According to Ayurveda

In our fast-paced and hectic modern lives, it's easy to overlook the profound impact that our food choices have on our well-being. Ayurveda, the ancient Indian system of medicine, teaches us the art of mindful eating and the importance of conscious food choices. Ayurvedic principles guide us to nourish our bodies and souls by honoring the connection between food, digestion, and overall health. In this article, we explore the wisdom of Ayurveda and delve into the transformative power of mindful eating and conscious food choices.

What is Mindful Eating?
Mindful eating is a practice rooted in awareness and presence. It invites us to slow down, engage our senses, and cultivate a deeper connection with our food. Rather than mindlessly consuming meals, we become fully present and attentive to the experience of eating. By savoring each bite, we develop a profound appreciation for the nourishment that food provides.

The Importance of Conscious Food Choices
Ayurveda recognizes that food is not just a source of physical sustenance but also a powerful form of medicine. The choices we make regarding what we eat directly impact our physical, mental, and emotional well-being.

Ayurveda categorizes foods based on their qualities and effects on the doshas (Vata, Pitta, and Kapha). By understanding our unique constitution and the needs of our body, we can make conscious food choices that promote balance and harmony within.

Eating According to the Doshas

Ayurveda teaches us that each person has a unique doshic constitution. Vata types benefit from warm, nourishing, and grounding foods, Pitta types thrive on cooling and calming foods, while Kapha types require light and stimulating foods. By aligning our diet with our dosha, we can support our body's innate intelligence and maintain a state of equilibrium.

The Six Tastes

Ayurveda recognizes six tastes: sweet, sour, salty, pungent, bitter, and astringent. Each taste has distinct qualities and effects on the doshas. Including a variety of tastes in our meals ensures that we receive a balanced spectrum of nutrients and promotes overall well-being. For example, the sweet taste nourishes and grounds Vata, while the bitter taste helps balance Pitta. By incorporating all six tastes, we can create meals that are satisfying and nutritionally balanced.

Honoring the Digestive Fire

Ayurveda places great emphasis on Agni, the digestive fire responsible for breaking down food and assimilating nutrients. To support optimal digestion, it's important to eat in a calm and relaxed environment, free from distractions. Additionally, Ayurveda recommends consuming foods that are easily digestible and properly cooked to avoid straining the digestive system.

Cultivating Gratitude and Connection

Mindful eating is not just about the physical act of consuming food but also about cultivating gratitude and connection with our meals. Ayurveda encourages us to appreciate the journey that our food takes from seed to plate, recognizing the efforts of farmers, cooks, and nature itself. By acknowledging the interconnectedness of all beings, we develop a deeper reverence for the nourishment that sustains us.

Bringing Mindful Eating into Practice

To embrace the art of mindful eating, start by setting aside dedicated time for meals, free from distractions like screens or work. Engage your senses by observing the colors, aromas, textures, and flavors of your food. Chew slowly and thoroughly, allowing the digestive enzymes in your saliva to break down the food. Tune into your body's signals of hunger and satiety, eating until you feel comfortably satisfied rather than overindulging.

Incorporate conscious food choices by selecting fresh, seasonal, and organic ingredients whenever possible. Opt for whole, unprocessed foods that are in harmony with your dosha. Listen to your body's wisdom and choose foods that leave you feeling energized and balanced.

By embracing the art of mindful eating and making conscious food choices, we can transform our relationship with food. We not only nourish our bodies but also honor the profound connection between food and our overall well-being. Let us embark on this journey of mindful eating, cultivating a deeper sense of gratitude, harmony, and vitality in our lives.

The Six Tastes and Their Effects on the Doshas: Balancing Body and Mind Through Ayurvedic Wisdom

In Ayurveda, the ancient Indian system of medicine, food is not just a source of physical nourishment, but also a powerful tool for maintaining balance and promoting optimal health. According to Ayurveda, there are six tastes, each with its own unique qualities and effects on the doshas (Vata, Pitta, and Kapha). By understanding the characteristics of these tastes and their impact on the doshas, we can make conscious food choices that support our individual constitution and promote harmony within the body and mind. In this article, we explore the six tastes and their effects on the doshas, empowering us to create balanced and nourishing meals.

1. Sweet (Madhura):
The sweet taste is nourishing, grounding, and soothing. It helps pacify Vata and Pitta doshas, providing stability and comfort. Sweet foods include fruits, grains like rice and wheat, dairy products, honey, and sweet vegetables like carrots and sweet potatoes. However, it's important to consume sweet foods in moderation to prevent imbalances such as weight gain or sluggishness.

2. Sour (Amla):
The sour taste is refreshing, stimulating, and heating. It can aggravate Pitta and increase the production of digestive acids. Sour foods include citrus fruits, yogurt, fermented foods, and vinegar. When consumed in moderation, sour foods can support digestion and help balance Kapha. However, excessive consumption can lead to Pitta imbalances such as heartburn or acidity.

3. Salty (Lavana):
The salty taste is grounding, hydrating, and stimulating. It can aggravate

Pitta and Kapha doshas, so it's important to consume salty foods in moderation. Salty foods include sea salt, rock salt, seaweed, and salty cheeses. Salt is essential for proper electrolyte balance, but excessive intake can lead to fluid retention and increased blood pressure.

4. Pungent (Katu):

The pungent taste is heating, stimulating, and drying. It can aggravate Pitta and Vata doshas, so it's important to consume pungent foods in moderation. Pungent foods include spices like chili peppers, ginger, garlic, onions, and certain herbs. The pungent taste can improve digestion, enhance circulation, and clear congestion when used appropriately, but excessive intake can cause Pitta imbalances such as inflammation or irritability.

5. Bitter (Tikta):

The bitter taste is cooling, cleansing, and drying. It can help balance Pitta and Kapha doshas, but it may aggravate Vata when consumed excessively. Bitter foods include leafy greens, bitter melon, turmeric, fenugreek, and certain herbs. The bitter taste stimulates the liver, aids in detoxification, and promotes healthy digestion. However, its strong nature may not be suitable for everyone, especially those with Vata imbalances or low body weight.

6. Astringent (Kashaya):

The astringent taste is cooling, drying, and contracting. It can help balance Pitta and Kapha doshas, but it may increase Vata when consumed excessively. Astringent foods include legumes, pomegranates, green tea, and certain vegetables like cabbage and Brussels sprouts. The astringent taste can support healthy skin, promote tissue healing, and aid in managing excessive oiliness or moisture. However, it can also create dryness, so it's important to balance it with other tastes.

In Ayurvedic nutrition, a well-balanced meal should ideally contain all six tastes in appropriate proportions. This ensures that we receive a wide array of nutrients and maintain doshic balance. Each individual has a unique constitution, and understanding your doshic makeup can guide you in making conscious food choices that promote harmony and well-being.

Remember that Ayurveda emphasizes moderation and mindful eating. It's essential to listen to your body and observe how different tastes affect you personally. By incorporating the six tastes in your meals mindfully, you can support your doshic constitution, optimize digestion, and promote overall balance and vitality.

In conclusion, the six tastes offer a comprehensive framework for understanding the effects of food on the doshas. By consciously incorporating the sweet, sour, salty, pungent, bitter, and astringent tastes into our diet, we can create meals that nourish our bodies, balance our doshas, and support our overall well-being. Let this wisdom guide your food choices and empower you to embark on a journey of optimal health and vitality through the nourishing power of Ayurvedic nutrition.

Designing a Balanced Ayurvedic Diet for Your Constitution: Nourishing Your Unique Self

Ayurveda, the ancient Indian system of medicine, teaches us that each individual is unique and has a distinct constitution or doshic makeup. Understanding our doshic constitution (Vata, Pitta, or Kapha) is key to designing a balanced Ayurvedic diet that supports our overall well-being. By aligning our food choices with our constitutional needs, we can nurture our bodies, maintain harmony, and promote optimal health. In this article, we explore the principles of designing a balanced Ayurvedic diet for your constitution, empowering you to nourish your unique self.

Know Your Dosha

The first step in designing a balanced Ayurvedic diet is to determine your doshic constitution. This can be done through self-reflection or by consulting with an Ayurvedic practitioner who can assess your physical and psychological traits. Vata types tend to have qualities of air and space, Pitta types exhibit fire and water qualities, and Kapha types embody earth and water characteristics. Understanding your dominant dosha helps you make appropriate food choices that support your specific needs.

Balancing the Doshas

Once you know your doshic constitution, the aim is to create balance within your body by pacifying any excess dosha while nourishing the deficient dosha. For example, a Vata type, characterized by qualities of dryness, coldness, and mobility, benefits from warm, grounding, and nourishing foods to counterbalance these tendencies. Similarly, a Pitta type, with qualities of heat, intensity, and sharpness, can find balance by incorporating cooling and calming foods. And a Kapha type, with qualities of heaviness, coolness, and stability, benefits from light, stimulating, and warming foods.

General Guidelines for Each Dosha

While individual needs may vary, there are general guidelines that can help you design a balanced Ayurvedic diet for your constitution:

1. Vata-Pacifying Diet:
Focus on warm and cooked foods, including soups, stews, and steamed vegetables. Incorporate healthy fats like ghee and oils to nourish and moisturize. Opt for grounding grains like rice and quinoa, and favor sweet, sour, and salty tastes. Avoid excessive cold, raw, and dry foods, as well as stimulants like caffeine.

2. Pitta-Pacifying Diet:
Emphasize cooling and refreshing foods, such as fresh fruits and vegetables, cucumber, coconut, and cilantro. Include bitter and astringent tastes. Favor whole grains like basmati rice and barley. Minimize spicy and oily foods, as well as alcohol and caffeine. Opt for gentle cooking methods like steaming and boiling.

3. Kapha-Pacifying Diet:
Choose light and warming foods, such as steamed vegetables, spices, and legumes. Emphasize pungent, bitter, and astringent tastes. Include grains like quinoa and amaranth. Limit heavy and oily foods, as well as dairy products. Opt for moderate cooking methods like baking and sautéing.

Listen to Your Body
While understanding your doshic constitution is essential, it's equally important to listen to your body's signals and adjust your diet accordingly. Your needs may vary based on factors like season, age, and current imbalances. Pay attention to how different foods make you feel. Notice if certain foods aggravate or alleviate symptoms. Your body's intelligence will guide you towards making choices that promote balance and well-being.

Incorporate Mindful Eating Practices
In addition to food choices, Ayurveda emphasizes the practice of mindful eating. Slow down, savor each bite, and eat in a calm and relaxed environment. Avoid distractions like screens or work while eating. Chew your food thoroughly to support proper digestion. Cultivate gratitude for the nourishment your food provides and the effort that went into producing it.

Seek Guidance
Designing a balanced Ayurvedic diet can be a complex process, especially if you're new to Ayurveda. Consider seeking guidance from an Ayurvedic practitioner who can provide personalized recommendations based on your unique constitution, current health status, and specific goals.

In conclusion, designing a balanced Ayurvedic diet for your constitution is a holistic approach to nourishing your unique self. By aligning your food choices with your doshic makeup, you can promote balance, vitality, and overall well-being. Embrace the wisdom of Ayurveda, listen to your body, and cultivate a deeper connection with the food you consume. Let the healing power of a balanced Ayurvedic diet support you on your journey to optimal health and harmony.

Ayurvedic Cooking Methods and Spices for Therapeutic Benefits: Harnessing the Healing Power of Food

In Ayurveda, the ancient system of holistic healing, food is not merely seen as sustenance but as a powerful tool for promoting health and well-being. Ayurvedic cooking methods and the use of therapeutic spices are essential components of this approach. By understanding and incorporating these methods and spices into our culinary practices, we can enhance digestion, support the body's natural healing processes, and balance the doshas. In this article, we explore the art of Ayurvedic cooking and the therapeutic benefits of various cooking methods and spices.

Ayurvedic Cooking Methods:

Sautéing/Tempering (Tadka/Bharjana): Sautéing/Tempering is a common Ayurvedic cooking method that involves heating ghee or oil and adding spices to release their flavors and therapeutic properties. The heat helps enhance the digestibility of spices, making them more accessible to the body. Sautéing also infuses the dish with aromatic flavors, stimulating the senses and improving the overall dining experience.

Steaming (Svedana): Steaming is a gentle cooking method that preserves the nutritional value of food while making it easier to digest. It is particularly beneficial for Vata and Pitta types who may have sensitive digestive systems. Steamed vegetables, grains, and proteins retain their natural moisture, making them nourishing and gentle on the digestive tract.

Boiling (Pachana): Boiling is a simple and effective cooking method in Ayurveda. It is often used to prepare soups, stews, and herbal decoctions. Boiling helps break down the ingredients, making them easier to digest and extract their medicinal properties. This method is beneficial for balancing Kapha as it reduces heaviness and promotes warmth and lightness in the body.

Baking (Taapana): Baking is a dry heat cooking method that imparts a unique flavor to the ingredients. It is a preferred method for preparing grains, vegetables, and certain proteins. Baking helps retain the natural sweetness of the food while providing a crisp texture. It is a grounding method that balances Vata and adds warmth to the body.

Fermenting (Sandhana): Fermentation is a traditional Ayurvedic technique used to preserve and enhance the digestibility of certain foods. Fermented foods like yogurt, sauerkraut, and dosas (fermented rice pancakes) promote the growth of beneficial bacteria in the gut, supporting digestion and boosting immunity. They also help balance Vata and Kapha doshas.

Ayurvedic Spices:

1. Turmeric (Haridra):

Turmeric is a vibrant yellow spice with powerful anti-inflammatory and antioxidant properties. It supports digestion, detoxification, and joint health. Turmeric contains an active compound called curcumin, which has been extensively studied for its therapeutic benefits.

2. Cumin (Jeera):

Cumin seeds are widely used in Ayurvedic cooking for their digestive benefits. They stimulate the digestive fire (agni), improve nutrient absorption, and alleviate bloating and gas. Cumin also has a balancing effect on all three doshas.

3. Coriander (Dhania):

Coriander seeds and leaves are integral to Ayurvedic cuisine. They have cooling properties and aid in digestion. Coriander helps to balance Pitta dosha, promotes healthy metabolism, and adds a pleasant flavor to dishes.

4. Mustard Seeds (Sarson):

Mustard seeds are commonly used in Ayurvedic cooking for their pungent and heating properties. They stimulate digestion, improve appetite, and enhance the flavor of dishes. Mustard seeds also have antimicrobial properties, making them beneficial for overall health.

5. Hing (Asafoetida):

Hing, also known as asafoetida, is a resin derived from the Ferula plant. It has a strong aroma and a pungent flavor. In Ayurveda, hing is valued for its digestive properties and its ability to alleviate gas and bloating. It is commonly used in lentil dishes and vegetable preparations.

6. Fenugreek (Methi):

Fenugreek seeds are widely used in Ayurvedic cooking for their bitter taste and numerous health benefits. They support digestion, help balance blood sugar levels, and have a positive impact on respiratory health. Fenugreek seeds can be used in spice blends, curries, and herbal teas.

When using these Ayurvedic spices, it's important to consider their individual qualities and the needs of your doshic constitution. Balancing the six tastes (sweet, sour, salty, pungent, bitter, and astringent) in your meals is also crucial for maintaining doshic equilibrium and overall well-being.

In conclusion, Ayurvedic cooking methods and the use of therapeutic spices go beyond enhancing the flavors of our meals. They have a profound impact on our digestion, metabolism, and overall health. By incorporating these methods and spices into our daily cooking practices, we can create nourishing and balanced meals that support our unique doshic constitution. Embrace the wisdom of Ayurveda in your kitchen, and let the therapeutic benefits of Ayurvedic cooking enhance your well-being from within.

Ayurvedic Approaches to Fasting and Detoxification: Nurturing the Body, Mind, and Spirit

Fasting and detoxification have been practiced for centuries as a means to cleanse and rejuvenate the body. In Ayurveda, these practices hold significant importance for promoting optimal health and well-being. Ayurvedic approaches to fasting and detoxification focus not only on physical purification but also on balancing the doshas and nurturing the mind and spirit. In this article, we delve into the wisdom of Ayurveda and explore the principles and benefits of fasting and detoxification.

Understanding Fasting in Ayurveda:

Fasting, known as Upavasa in Ayurveda, involves abstaining from solid food or specific types of food for a designated period. It allows the digestive system to rest, promotes the elimination of toxins, and rekindles the body's natural healing mechanisms. Fasting can be practiced in various ways, such as intermittent fasting, juice fasting, or water fasting, depending on individual needs and preferences.

Benefits of Fasting in Ayurveda:

1. Detoxification and Cleansing: Fasting allows the body to eliminate accumulated toxins and waste products. It supports the detoxification process, improves digestion, and enhances the functioning of the liver and other eliminatory organs.

2. Rest and Regeneration: By giving the digestive system a break, fasting helps redirect energy towards cellular repair, rejuvenation, and healing. It promotes a sense of lightness, clarity, and vitality.

3. Balancing the Doshas: Fasting helps balance the doshas by reducing excesses and imbalances. It pacifies aggravated doshas and supports the restoration of doshic equilibrium, promoting overall health and well-being.

Ayurvedic Approaches to Detoxification:

1. Panchakarma:

Panchakarma is a comprehensive Ayurvedic detoxification and rejuvenation program. It involves a series of therapies, including herbal oil massages, steam treatments, and specialized detoxification procedures, tailored to individual needs. Panchakarma helps remove deep-seated toxins, rejuvenates the body, and restores balance to the doshas.

2. Dietary Detox:

Ayurveda emphasizes the importance of following a detoxifying diet to support the body's natural cleansing processes. This involves consuming light, easily digestible foods, such as kitchari (a blend of rice and lentils) and steamed vegetables, while avoiding processed foods, heavy meats, and refined sugars.

3. Herbal Support:

Ayurvedic herbs and formulations play a vital role in supporting detoxification. Triphala, a combination of three fruits, is a commonly used Ayurvedic herbal supplement known for its detoxifying properties. Other herbs like ginger, turmeric, and neem can also aid in the elimination of toxins and support overall detoxification.

Guidelines for Safe and Effective Fasting and Detoxification:

1. Individualization:

It's essential to consider your unique constitution (Prakriti), current health condition, and any imbalances or specific needs before embarking on a fasting or detoxification regimen. Seek guidance from an experienced Ayurvedic practitioner to ensure a personalized approach.

2. Preparation:

Before fasting or undergoing detoxification, it's important to prepare the body by gradually reducing heavy and processed foods, incorporating more fruits, vegetables, and whole grains, and staying well-hydrated. This helps ease the transition into fasting or a detox program.

3. Mindful Awareness:

Approach fasting and detoxification with a mindful and positive mindset. Take time for self-reflection, meditation, and gentle activities that nourish the mind and spirit. Practice self-care, deep breathing, and ensure adequate rest and relaxation.

4. Post-Detoxification Care:

After completing a fasting or detoxification program, it's crucial to reintroduce foods gradually and mindfully. Focus on wholesome, nourishing meals and continue to follow a balanced Ayurvedic diet and lifestyle to maintain the benefits achieved during the cleanse.

In conclusion, Ayurvedic approaches to fasting and detoxification offer a holistic and comprehensive way to support the body's natural healing and purification processes. By embracing these practices, we can experience physical rejuvenation, emotional well-being, and spiritual growth. However, it's important to approach fasting and detoxification with caution, seeking guidance from an Ayurvedic practitioner to ensure safety and efficacy. Let Ayurveda be your guide on this transformative journey of cleansing, renewal, and self-discovery.

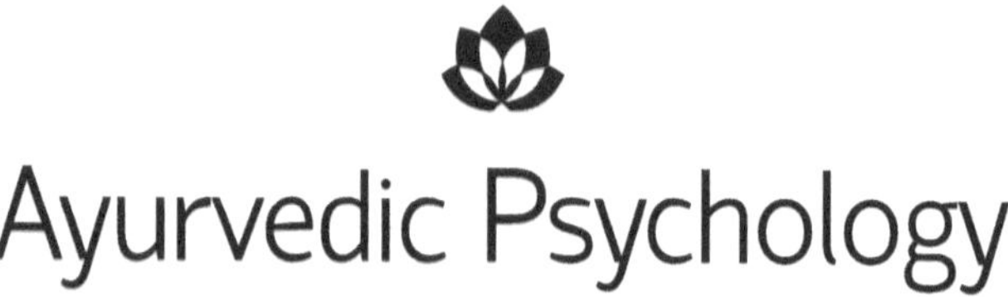

Ayurvedic Psychology

- Understanding the mind-body connection
- The impact of emotions and mental states on health
- Ayurvedic practices for stress reduction and relaxation
- Meditation and mindfulness techniques for emotional well-being
- Developing a positive mindset and cultivating self-awareness

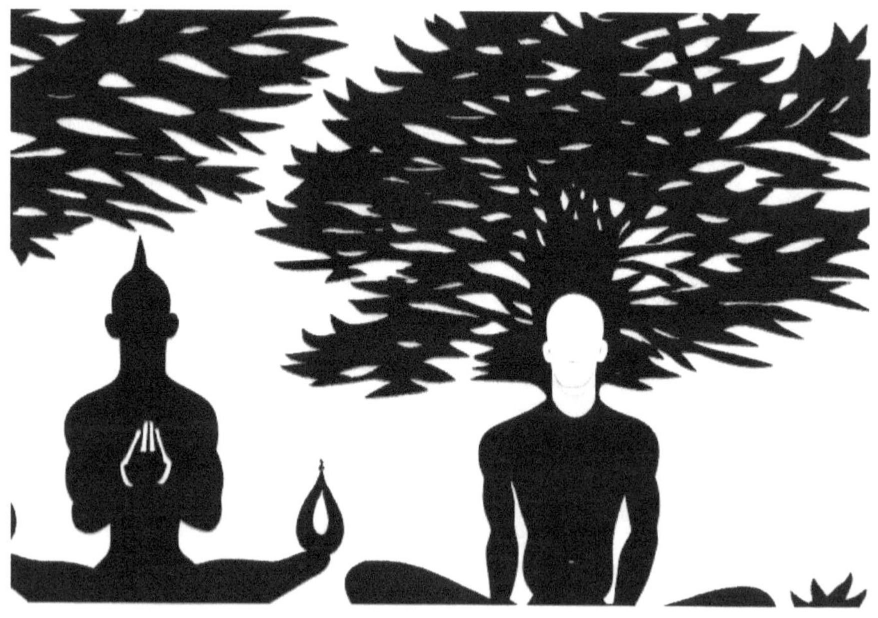

Mind Matters!

In Ayurveda, the ancient science of holistic healing, the mind and body are regarded as inseparable entities, with each profoundly influencing the other. Ayurvedic psychology delves into the intricate interplay between our mental states, emotions, and physical health, recognizing the vital role they play in achieving overall well-being. This branch of Ayurveda offers profound insights and practical tools to cultivate a harmonious mind-body connection and promote emotional balance. In this article, we explore the fundamental principles of Ayurvedic psychology and discover the transformative practices it offers.

Ayurvedic psychology emphasizes the importance of cultivating a positive mindset and developing self-awareness. This involves consciously choosing thoughts that support our well-being, practicing gratitude, engaging in positive affirmations, and reframing negative beliefs. Developing self-awareness helps us understand our emotions, triggers, and patterns, empowering us to respond rather than react to life's challenges.

Ayurvedic psychology invites us to explore the intricate relationship between our thoughts, emotions, and physical health. By nurturing the mind-body connection, incorporating stress-reducing practices, embracing meditation and mindfulness, and cultivating a positive mindset, we can embark on a transformative journey of self-discovery and holistic well-being. Ayurvedic psychology offers a comprehensive approach to nurturing our mental and emotional health, ultimately supporting our overall vitality and happiness.

Understanding the Mind-Body Connection: Exploring Ayurvedic Psychology

In Ayurveda, the ancient system of holistic healing, the mind and body are intricately interconnected. Ayurvedic psychology recognizes that our mental and emotional well-being significantly influences our physical health and vice versa. This perspective emphasizes the importance of understanding and nurturing the mind-body connection to achieve optimal health and balance. In this article, we delve into the principles of Ayurvedic psychology and explore the profound relationship between the mind and body.

The Three Doshas and Mental Constitution:

According to Ayurveda, each individual has a unique mind-body constitution, known as Prakriti, which is determined by the predominance of the three doshas—Vata, Pitta, and Kapha. These doshas not only influence our physical traits but also shape our mental and emotional characteristics. Understanding our Prakriti helps us gain insight into our natural tendencies, strengths, and areas of vulnerability from a psychological perspective.

Vata:

Individuals with a dominant Vata constitution tend to have a creative and active mind. They are often quick-thinking, imaginative, and prone to anxiety or worry when imbalanced. Balancing practices for Vata types involve cultivating stability, routine, and grounding activities such as meditation, gentle exercise, and calming herbs like ashwagandha.

Pitta:

Pitta-dominant individuals are known for their sharp intellect, ambition, and strong sense of purpose. However, imbalanced Pitta can lead to anger, irritability, and perfectionism. Pitta types benefit from practices that promote relaxation, moderation, and cooling of the mind, such as meditation, mindfulness, and incorporating cooling herbs like coriander.

Kapha:

Kapha types are characterized by their calmness, stability, and nurturing nature. However, when imbalanced, they may experience attachment, lethargy, and resistance to change. Invigorating practices that stimulate the mind and body, such as dynamic yoga, vigorous exercise, and energizing herbs like ginger, can help balance Kapha.

The Mind-Body Connection:

Ayurvedic psychology recognizes that our thoughts, emotions, and experiences have a direct impact on our physical health. Negative emotions, stress, and unresolved psychological issues can manifest as physical symptoms and imbalances in the body. Conversely, physical health issues can affect our mental and emotional well-being. This mind-body connection underscores the need to address both aspects to achieve true healing and well-being.

Ayurvedic Approaches to Balancing the Mind and Body:

1. Meditation and Mindfulness:

Practicing meditation and mindfulness cultivates awareness, stillness, and a deeper connection to the present moment. These practices help calm the mind, reduce stress, and promote overall mental and physical balance.

2. Ayurvedic Lifestyle:

Following an Ayurvedic lifestyle, tailored to your Prakriti, supports the mind-body connection. This includes maintaining a regular daily routine (Dinacharya), practicing self-care, eating balanced meals according to your constitution, and engaging in appropriate exercise and movement.

3. Sattvic Diet:

A sattvic diet is a vital aspect of Ayurvedic psychology as it promotes clarity, purity, and harmony of the mind. This diet consists of fresh, organic, and whole foods, including fruits, vegetables, whole grains, and light dairy products. It avoids processed, heavy, and overly stimulating foods.

4. Herbal Support:

Ayurveda utilizes specific herbs and herbal formulations to support mental and emotional well-being. Adaptogenic herbs like ashwagandha, brahmi, and shatavari are known for their ability to nourish the nervous system, enhance cognitive function, and promote emotional balance.

5. Emotional Release Techniques:

Emotional release techniques, such as journaling, counseling, and energy-based therapies like Ayurvedic marma therapy or acupuncture, can help release emotional blockages and promote healing on a deep psychological level.

By embracing the principles of Ayurvedic psychology, we can foster a harmonious mind-body connection and achieve holistic well-being. Recognizing our unique Prakriti and understanding the interplay between our thoughts, emotions, and physical health empowers us to make conscious choices that support our overall balance and vitality. Let Ayurveda be your guide in cultivating a deeper understanding of the mind-body connection and nurturing your holistic well-being.

The Impact of Emotions and Mental States on Health: Insights from Ayurvedic Psychology

In Ayurvedic psychology, the impact of emotions and mental states on our overall health is recognized as profound and interconnected. Ayurveda views the mind and body as inseparable entities, with each influencing the other in a dynamic and intricate manner. Emotions, thoughts, and mental states are seen as powerful forces that can either support or disrupt our well-being. By understanding and addressing the impact of these factors, Ayurvedic psychology offers valuable insights for promoting holistic health and balance. In this article, we explore the profound relationship between emotions, mental states, and our physical well-being within the framework of Ayurvedic psychology.

Emotions as Energy in Motion:

Ayurvedic psychology recognizes emotions as energetic experiences that affect the flow of vital energy (prana) within the body. When emotions are experienced and expressed harmoniously, they contribute to overall balance and well-being. However, unprocessed or repressed emotions can create energetic blockages, leading to imbalances and disturbances in the mind and body. Ayurveda emphasizes the importance of understanding, acknowledging, and effectively processing emotions to maintain optimal health.

The Role of Doshas in Emotional Well-being:

According to Ayurveda, our unique mind-body constitution, or Prakriti, is determined by the balance of the three doshas—Vata, Pitta, and Kapha. Each dosha is associated with specific emotional tendencies and responses. Imbalances in the doshas can contribute to the manifestation of emotional disturbances. For example:

1. Vata Imbalance: Excessive Vata can lead to anxiety, fear, restlessness, and emotional instability. On the other hand, when Vata is balanced, it promotes creativity, adaptability, and joy.

2. Pitta Imbalance: Imbalanced Pitta can manifest as anger, irritability, frustration, and critical tendencies. In a balanced state, Pitta fosters courage, intelligence, and a sense of purpose.

3. Kapha Imbalance: Imbalanced Kapha may result in attachment, lethargy, depression, and resistance to change. When Kapha is balanced, it promotes compassion, stability, and emotional grounding.

Addressing Emotions for Optimal Health:

Ayurvedic psychology offers practical approaches for addressing emotions and mental states to support optimal health and well-being:

1. Self-awareness: Developing self-awareness is crucial in recognizing and understanding our emotional patterns, triggers, and reactions. By observing our emotions without judgment, we can gain insights into the underlying causes and take appropriate steps towards healing and transformation.

2. Emotional Release: Ayurvedic therapies like Ayurvedic massage, yoga, pranayama (breathing exercises), and meditation provide avenues for emotional release and promoting energetic balance. These practices help release stagnant emotions, calm the mind, and create space for positive emotional experiences.

3. Herbal Support: Ayurveda utilizes specific herbs and formulations known for their positive effects on the mind and emotions. Adaptogenic herbs like ashwagandha, brahmi, and shatavari can help reduce anxiety, support emotional stability, and promote overall well-being.

4. Lifestyle Modifications: Ayurvedic psychology emphasizes the importance of cultivating a balanced lifestyle. This includes following a nurturing daily routine, eating a wholesome and balanced diet, engaging in appropriate exercise, practicing relaxation techniques, and nurturing healthy relationships.

By addressing and transforming our emotions and mental states, we can support the harmonious functioning of our mind and body, fostering overall health and well-being. Ayurvedic psychology invites us to develop a deep understanding of the interplay between our emotions, mental states, and physical health, empowering us to take proactive steps towards emotional balance, inner harmony, and holistic wellness.

Ayurvedic Practices for Stress Reduction and Relaxation: Nurturing Inner Harmony through Ayurvedic Psychology

In the fast-paced and demanding world we live in, stress has become an increasingly common concern affecting our physical and mental well-being. Ayurvedic psychology offers profound insights and practical tools for managing and reducing stress, fostering relaxation, and restoring balance. By incorporating Ayurvedic practices into our daily lives, we can nurture inner harmony, promote overall well-being, and navigate the challenges of modern life with greater ease. In this article, we explore the Ayurvedic approaches to stress reduction and relaxation within the framework of Ayurvedic psychology.

Understanding the Impact of Stress:

Stress, in Ayurveda, is seen as an imbalance that disrupts the natural harmony of the mind and body. It can arise from various sources, including work pressures, relationship challenges, financial worries, and lifestyle factors. When stress becomes chronic or overwhelming, it can lead to physical, mental, and emotional imbalances, compromising our overall health and vitality. Ayurvedic psychology recognizes the importance of managing stress to maintain optimal well-being.

Ayurvedic Practices for Stress Reduction and Relaxation:

1. Daily Routine (Dinacharya): Establishing a balanced daily routine is a fundamental aspect of Ayurvedic lifestyle. Consistency in waking up and sleeping times, meal timings, and daily self-care practices helps create stability, reduce stress, and promote relaxation. A well-structured routine nourishes the body and mind, providing a sense of grounding and support amidst the chaos of daily life.

2. Meditation and Mindfulness: These practices are integral to Ayurvedic psychology for managing stress. Meditation involves quieting the mind and directing our focus inward, cultivating a sense of calm and mental clarity. Mindfulness encourages us to be fully present in the moment, observing our thoughts and emotions without judgment. Regular practice of meditation and mindfulness helps reduce stress, improve resilience, and enhance overall well-being.

3. Abhyanga (Ayurvedic Self-Massage): Abhyanga is a self-massage technique using warm herbal oils that nourishes the body, calms the nervous system, and promotes relaxation. The rhythmic application of oil enhances circulation, soothes the mind, and releases stored tension. Practicing Abhyanga regularly is a powerful way to reduce stress and rejuvenate both the body and mind.

4. Yoga and Pranayama (Breathing Exercises): Yoga and pranayama practices are deeply rooted in Ayurveda and offer profound benefits for stress reduction. The gentle movements, stretching, and breath control in yoga help release physical and mental tension, promote relaxation, and balance the nervous system. Pranayama techniques, such as alternate nostril breathing or deep belly breathing, calm the mind and activate the body's relaxation response.

5. Herbal Support: Ayurveda harnesses the healing power of herbs to support stress reduction and relaxation. Adaptogenic herbs like ashwagandha, brahmi, and tulsi are known for their ability to nourish the nervous system, reduce anxiety, and promote a sense of calm. These herbs can be consumed in the form of herbal teas, herbal supplements, or as part of Ayurvedic formulations prescribed by an Ayurvedic practitioner.

6. Ayurvedic Therapies: Ayurvedic therapies such as Shirodhara (oil pouring on the forehead), Panchakarma (detoxification treatments), and Ayurvedic massages (like Marma therapy) are highly effective in reducing stress, releasing physical and mental tension, and promoting deep relaxation. These therapies are best administered by trained Ayurvedic practitioners to ensure their safe and appropriate application.

7. Nurturing Self-Care: Practicing self-care is vital for managing stress and promoting relaxation. This may include engaging in activities that bring joy and nourishment, such as spending time in nature, engaging in creative pursuits, cultivating healthy relationships, and setting aside time for hobbies or relaxation practices like listening to soothing music or taking a warm bath.

By incorporating these Ayurvedic practices into our daily lives, we can proactively manage stress, promote relaxation, and foster a sense of inner harmony. Ayurvedic psychology recognizes the importance of nurturing our overall well-being, not just treating the symptoms of stress. Through these practices, we can cultivate resilience, enhance our ability to adapt to life's challenges, and maintain a state of balance and tranquility amidst the demands of our modern world.

Meditation and Mindfulness Techniques for Emotional Well-being: Cultivating Inner Balance with Ayurvedic Psychology

In the realm of Ayurvedic psychology, meditation and mindfulness practices hold a significant place in nurturing emotional well-being. These powerful techniques offer profound benefits for managing and transforming emotions, reducing stress, and fostering inner peace and harmony. By incorporating meditation and mindfulness into our daily lives, we can develop a deeper understanding of our emotions, cultivate a positive mindset, and navigate the ups and downs of life with greater equanimity. In this article, we explore the transformative role of meditation and mindfulness within the framework of Ayurvedic psychology.

Understanding Meditation and Mindfulness:

Meditation is a practice that involves training the mind to focus and redirect its thoughts, ultimately leading to a state of mental clarity and emotional balance. Mindfulness, on the other hand, is the practice of being fully present in the moment, observing our thoughts, emotions, and sensations without judgment. Both meditation and mindfulness serve as gateways to self-awareness, providing an opportunity to explore the intricate landscape of our inner world.

Cultivating Emotional Well-being:

1. Embracing Present-Moment Awareness: The practice of mindfulness invites us to anchor our attention in the present moment, allowing us to fully experience and acknowledge our emotions without getting caught up

in them. By observing our emotions with non-judgmental awareness, we can develop a deeper understanding of their transient nature and learn to respond to them with greater compassion and wisdom.

2. Developing Emotional Resilience: Regular meditation and mindfulness practice strengthen our capacity to navigate challenging emotions. By creating a space of stillness and non-reactivity, we can observe emotions as they arise, understanding their underlying causes and allowing them to naturally dissipate. This cultivates emotional resilience, enabling us to respond to situations with clarity and composure rather than being overwhelmed by our emotions.

3. Transforming Negative Thought Patterns: Meditation and mindfulness help us become aware of recurring negative thought patterns that contribute to emotional distress. Through focused attention and gentle inquiry, we can challenge and reframe these patterns, replacing them with more positive and empowering thoughts. This shift in thinking supports emotional well-being and helps us cultivate a positive mindset.

4. Cultivating Compassion and Self-Compassion: Meditation and mindfulness practices encourage us to cultivate compassion, both for ourselves and others. As we develop a deep sense of self-awareness and understanding, we can extend kindness and compassion to ourselves when faced with difficult emotions. This self-compassion creates a foundation for emotional healing and promotes a sense of inner safety and well-being.

5. Cultivating Equanimity: The regular practice of meditation and mindfulness fosters a sense of equanimity—a balanced and non-reactive state of mind. By observing the ever-changing nature of our thoughts and emotions, we develop a greater sense of detachment and acceptance. This equanimity allows us to ride the waves of emotions with grace, remaining steady and centered amidst the storms of life.

Incorporating Meditation and Mindfulness into Daily Life:

1. Set aside dedicated time for meditation and mindfulness practice. Start with just a few minutes each day and gradually increase the duration as you become more comfortable.

2. Find a quiet and peaceful space where you can practice without distractions.

3. Experiment with different meditation techniques such as breath awareness, loving-kindness meditation, or guided visualizations to find what resonates with you.

4. Practice mindfulness throughout the day by bringing awareness to daily activities like eating, walking, or engaging in conversations. Fully engage your senses in the present moment.

5. Consider attending meditation or mindfulness retreats or workshops to deepen your practice and connect with like-minded individuals.

By integrating meditation and mindfulness into our daily lives, we can develop a profound sense of self-awareness, cultivate emotional well-being, and nurture inner balance. Ayurvedic psychology acknowledges the crucial role of these practices in transforming our relationship with emotions and promoting a state of inner harmony. As we embark on this journey of self-discovery, may we find solace, wisdom, and deep healing through the practice of meditation and mindfulness.

Developing a Positive Mindset and Cultivating Self-Awareness: Nurturing Inner Growth through Ayurvedic Psychology

In the realm of Ayurvedic psychology, developing a positive mindset and cultivating self-awareness are fundamental pillars for personal growth, emotional well-being, and overall balance. Ayurveda recognizes the profound impact of our thoughts, beliefs, and perceptions on our health, happiness, and quality of life. By consciously cultivating a positive mindset and nurturing self-awareness, we can transform our inner landscape, embrace our true potential, and lead a more fulfilling and purposeful life. In this article, we explore the significance of developing a positive mindset and cultivating self-awareness within the framework of Ayurvedic psychology.

Understanding the Power of the Mind:

Ayurvedic psychology recognizes that our minds are powerful instruments that shape our experiences, perceptions, and responses to life. The quality of our thoughts and beliefs directly influences our emotions, behaviors, and overall well-being. By becoming aware of the mind-body connection, we can harness the power of our thoughts to create positive shifts in our lives.

Cultivating a Positive Mindset:

1. Practicing Gratitude: Gratitude is a transformative practice that shifts our focus from what is lacking to what is present in our lives. By cultivating gratitude, we develop a positive outlook and foster a deep appreciation for the blessings and abundance around us. Regularly expressing gratitude can

uplift our mood, improve our relationships, and enhance our overall well-being.

2. Affirmations and Positive Self-Talk: Affirmations are powerful statements that reinforce positive beliefs and attitudes. By consciously choosing and repeating affirmations, we can reprogram our subconscious mind and cultivate a positive self-image. Positive self-talk involves replacing negative self-criticism with supportive and encouraging inner dialogue, fostering self-compassion and self-empowerment.

3. Embracing Optimism: Optimism is the mindset of seeing opportunities in challenges and maintaining a positive perspective in the face of adversity. By reframing negative situations, focusing on solutions rather than problems, and cultivating a sense of hope, we can develop resilience, reduce stress, and foster a positive mindset.

4. Surrounding Yourself with Positive Influences: Our environment and the people we surround ourselves with significantly impact our mindset. Surrounding ourselves with positive influences, supportive relationships, and uplifting communities can inspire and motivate us, reinforcing our positive mindset and fostering personal growth.

Cultivating Self-Awareness:

1. Reflection and Self-Inquiry: Self-awareness begins with self-reflection and self-inquiry. Take time to introspect, observe your thoughts and emotions, and explore the patterns and beliefs that shape your experiences. This process of self-inquiry helps uncover deep-rooted patterns, limiting beliefs, and areas for personal growth.

2. Mindfulness and Observation: Mindfulness practices, such as meditation and conscious breathing, cultivate present-moment awareness and enhance self-awareness. By observing our thoughts, emotions, and sensations without judgment, we develop a deeper understanding of ourselves and gain clarity about our desires, values, and aspirations.

3. Journaling and Self-Expression: Journaling is a powerful tool for self-reflection and self-expression. By writing down your thoughts, feelings, and experiences, you can gain insights, uncover patterns, and track your personal growth journey. Journaling provides a safe space to explore and express yourself authentically.

4. Seek Guidance and Support: Sometimes, cultivating self-awareness requires external guidance. Working with an Ayurvedic practitioner, therapist, or coach can provide valuable insights and support on your journey of self-discovery. They can help you navigate challenges, explore

limiting beliefs, and develop strategies for personal growth and positive transformation.

By consciously cultivating a positive mindset and nurturing self-awareness, we take ownership of our thoughts, beliefs, and emotions. In doing so, we empower ourselves to navigate life's challenges with resilience, embrace our true potential, and live a more fulfilling and purposeful existence. Ayurvedic psychology reminds us that our minds are potent tools for personal transformation, and by harnessing their power, we can create a life of joy, abundance, and inner harmony.

CHAPTER SIX

Ayurvedic Beauty and Self-Care

- Nurturing the body through Ayurvedic self-care rituals (Abhyanga, Neti, etc.)
- Ayurvedic skincare and natural beauty remedies
- Hair and scalp care using Ayurvedic principles
- Ayurvedic practices for maintaining oral health
- Ayurvedic approaches to aging gracefully

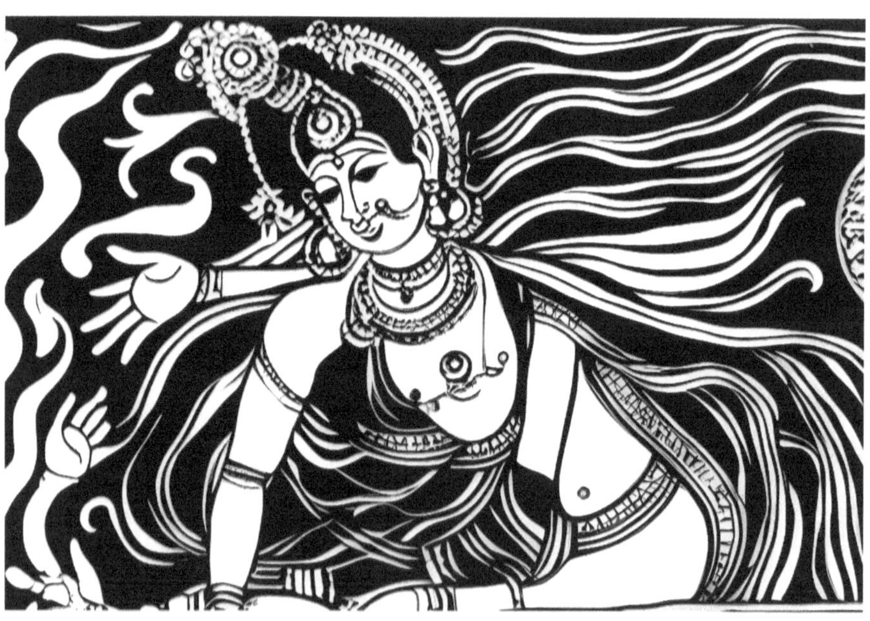

Ayurveda & Beauty

In the realm of Ayurveda, beauty is viewed as a reflection of inner well-being and balance. Ayurvedic beauty and self-care practices encompass a holistic approach to nurturing both our inner and outer radiance. Rooted in ancient wisdom and natural remedies, Ayurveda offers a treasure trove of rituals and principles to enhance our beauty, promote self-care, and support overall well-being. In this article, we explore the essence of Ayurvedic beauty and self-care, including nurturing the body through self-care rituals, skincare and natural beauty remedies, hair and scalp care, maintaining oral health, and aging gracefully.

As we dive into the world of Ayurvedic beauty and self-care, we embark on a journey that celebrates our unique beauty, supports our well-being, and nurtures our mind, body, and spirit. By incorporating these ancient practices and principles into our daily lives, we can experience the transformative power of Ayurveda and cultivate a radiant inner and outer beauty that radiates from within.

Nurturing the Body through Ayurvedic Self-Care Rituals: Embracing Holistic Well-being

In the ancient science of Ayurveda, self-care rituals play a vital role in nurturing and maintaining optimal health and well-being. These rituals are designed to nourish the body, balance the doshas (energetic forces), and promote a harmonious mind-body connection. By incorporating Ayurvedic self-care practices into our daily routines, we can cultivate self-love, enhance vitality, and experience a profound sense of rejuvenation. In this article, we explore some of the key Ayurvedic self-care rituals that nurture the body and support holistic well-being.

1. Abhyanga (Self-Massage): Abhyanga is a sacred self-massage practice using warm herbal oils. It is not only a deeply relaxing ritual but also a powerful way to nourish the skin, improve circulation, and promote detoxification. The rhythmic strokes of self-massage help balance the doshas, calm the nervous system, and provide a loving connection with our bodies. It is recommended to use dosha-specific oils, such as sesame oil for Vata, coconut or sunflower oil for Pitta, and almond or olive oil for Kapha.

2. Neti (Nasal Cleansing): Neti is a cleansing technique that involves rinsing the nasal passages with warm saline water. It helps remove

accumulated mucus, dust, and allergens, while soothing and moisturizing the nasal passages. Neti is particularly beneficial for those with sinus congestion, allergies, or respiratory issues. Using a neti pot or a saline nasal spray, practice this ritual regularly to promote clear breathing and maintain the health of the respiratory system.

3. Tongue Scraping: Tongue scraping is a simple yet effective Ayurvedic practice to remove toxins and bacteria from the tongue. By gently scraping the surface of the tongue with a copper or stainless-steel tongue scraper, we eliminate ama (toxic buildup) and enhance oral hygiene. This practice also stimulates the taste buds, promotes digestion, and freshens breath. Make tongue scraping a part of your daily oral care routine, ideally in the morning before brushing your teeth.

4. Dry Brushing (Garshana): Dry brushing is a traditional Ayurvedic technique that involves using a natural bristle brush to gently exfoliate the skin. The rhythmic brushing motion stimulates the lymphatic system, improves circulation, and helps remove dead skin cells. Dry brushing also enhances detoxification, promotes a healthy glow, and supports the overall health of the skin. Before showering, use a dry brush and gently stroke your body in upward motions, starting from the feet and moving towards the heart.

5. Oil Pulling: Oil pulling is an Ayurvedic practice that involves swishing oil in the mouth for 10-15 minutes to remove toxins and promote oral health. Traditionally, sesame or coconut oil is used for oil pulling. This practice helps remove bacteria, supports gum health, reduces bad breath, and can even contribute to overall detoxification. Remember to spit out the oil after oil pulling and rinse your mouth thoroughly with water.

6. Herbal Baths: Herbal baths are a delightful way to relax, rejuvenate, and nourish the body. Adding Ayurvedic herbs, such as rose petals, lavender, neem leaves, or chamomile, to your bathwater infuses it with therapeutic properties. These herbs can help calm the mind, soothe the skin, relieve muscle tension, and promote overall well-being. Enjoy a warm herbal bath regularly as part of your self-care routine.

7. Daily Rituals: Alongside specific self-care practices, Ayurveda emphasizes the importance of daily rituals to honor and nurture the body. These rituals include waking up early in the

morning, practicing yoga or gentle stretches, practicing pranayama (breathing exercises), drinking warm water with lemon, sipping herbal teas throughout the day, eating mindfully, and winding down with a relaxing bedtime routine. These daily rituals create a sense of rhythm and balance, supporting the body's natural healing processes.

By embracing these Ayurvedic self-care rituals, we honor our bodies as sacred vessels and create a foundation for holistic well-being. Incorporate these practices into your daily routine with mindfulness, intention, and self-love, and experience the transformative power of Ayurvedic self-care in nurturing and revitalizing your body, mind, and spirit.

Ayurvedic Skincare and Natural Beauty Remedies: Unlocking Radiance from Within

In the pursuit of beauty and radiance, Ayurveda offers a holistic approach that emphasizes nurturing the skin, restoring balance, and promoting overall well-being. Ayurvedic skincare and natural beauty remedies harness the power of nature, using time-tested herbs, oils, and ingredients to enhance our skin's health and vitality. Rooted in ancient wisdom and tailored to individual dosha types, Ayurvedic beauty rituals provide a transformative and sustainable path to radiant skin. In this article, we delve into the world of Ayurvedic skincare and explore the natural beauty remedies that can unlock your inner glow.

Understanding Ayurvedic Skincare:

Ayurvedic skincare revolves around the concept of balancing the doshas (Vata, Pitta, and Kapha) to maintain skin health and harmony. Each dosha has unique characteristics that influence our skin type and its specific needs. By understanding our dosha type, we can choose the most suitable skincare practices and products that address our skin concerns effectively.

Cleansing and Purifying:

In Ayurveda, cleansing the skin is not only about removing dirt and impurities but also about nourishing and balancing the skin. Herbal cleansers like besan (gram flour), rose water, and neem powder are gentle yet effective in purifying the skin without stripping away its natural oils. These natural ingredients help remove toxins, unclog pores, and promote a clear and radiant complexion.

Exfoliation and Detoxification:

Exfoliation plays a crucial role in Ayurvedic skincare by eliminating dead skin cells, improving circulation, and enhancing the skin's natural radiance. Ayurvedic exfoliants like ubtan (a paste made with herbs, grains, and oils) or finely ground herbs such as sandalwood, turmeric, and fenugreek can be used to gently slough off dead skin cells, leaving the skin soft, smooth, and glowing.

Nourishment and Moisturization:

Ayurvedic beauty emphasizes the importance of providing nourishment and hydration to the skin. Herbal oils such as almond oil, coconut oil, or sesame oil are commonly used to moisturize and rejuvenate the skin. These oils deeply penetrate the skin, restoring moisture, improving elasticity, and promoting a youthful complexion. Ayurvedic facial oils infused with specific herbs and botanicals can also target specific skin concerns such as dryness, inflammation, or hyperpigmentation.

Face Masks and Herbal Packs:

Ayurvedic face masks and herbal packs are potent remedies that harness the healing properties of herbs, fruits, and other natural ingredients. Ingredients like turmeric, sandalwood, rose petals, aloe vera, and multani mitti (Fuller's earth) are commonly used to create masks that address various skin concerns. These masks help cleanse, tone, tighten, and rejuvenate the skin, revealing a refreshed and radiant complexion.

Eye Care:

The delicate skin around the eyes requires special attention and care. Ayurvedic remedies like cucumber slices, rose water, or nourishing herbal eye creams can help reduce puffiness, dark circles, and fine lines. These remedies soothe and rejuvenate the eye area, providing a refreshed and youthful appearance.

Lip Care:

To keep the lips soft, supple, and hydrated, Ayurveda recommends using natural ingredients such as ghee, honey, or almond oil. These natural remedies nourish and moisturize the lips, preventing dryness, chapping, and promoting natural lip color.

Incorporating Ayurvedic beauty remedies into your skincare routine allows you to embrace a more holistic and natural approach to self-care. These remedies work in harmony with your body's innate healing capabilities, promoting overall well-being while enhancing your skin's health and radiance. Remember to choose products and practices that align with your dosha type and listen to your skin's unique needs. By unlocking the power of Ayurvedic skincare, you can unveil the timeless beauty that resides within you.

Hair and Scalp Care: Unveiling the Secrets of Ayurvedic Principles

In the realm of Ayurveda, the hair is considered a crown of beauty and vitality. Healthy and lustrous hair not only enhances our appearance but also reflects our overall well-being. Ayurvedic principles provide a comprehensive and holistic approach to hair and scalp care, focusing on nourishment, balance, and natural remedies. By embracing these principles, we can unlock the secrets to vibrant, strong, and beautiful hair. In this article, we delve into the world of Ayurvedic hair and scalp care, exploring the principles, practices, and natural remedies that can transform your hair care routine.

Understanding Hair and Scalp from an Ayurvedic Perspective:

According to Ayurveda, our hair type and its condition are influenced by the doshas (Vata, Pitta, and Kapha) and the balance or imbalance within them. Each dosha has specific characteristics that manifest in our hair, determining its texture, thickness, and susceptibility to various hair concerns. By understanding our dominant dosha and its impact on our hair, we can tailor our hair care practices to maintain balance and promote optimal hair health.

Scalp Nourishment and Cleansing:

A healthy scalp forms the foundation for vibrant hair. Ayurveda emphasizes the importance of maintaining a clean and nourished scalp to support healthy hair growth. Regular oil massages, known as Abhyanga, are integral to Ayurvedic hair care. Massaging the scalp with warm herbal oils like coconut oil, brahmi oil, or amla oil nourishes the roots, improves blood circulation, and promotes relaxation. These oils penetrate deeply, strengthening the hair follicles, preventing dryness, and reducing scalp-related concerns.

Herbal Cleansers and Shampoos:

Ayurvedic hair care encourages the use of natural and gentle cleansers that are free from harsh chemicals. Herbal powders like shikakai, reetha (soapnuts), and amla are popular alternatives to commercial shampoos. These natural cleansers cleanse the scalp, remove impurities, and promote healthy hair growth without stripping away the hair's natural oils. They also help maintain the pH balance of the scalp, preventing excessive dryness or oiliness.

Conditioning and Nourishing:

Ayurveda emphasizes the use of natural ingredients to condition and nourish the hair. Herbal rinses and hair masks prepared from ingredients like aloe vera, hibiscus, fenugreek, and yogurt provide deep conditioning, repair damaged hair, and add luster and strength. Ayurvedic hair oils enriched with herbs such as bhringraj, brahmi, and henna are also beneficial for promoting hair growth, preventing hair fall, and maintaining healthy hair.

Scalp Exfoliation and Detoxification:

Similar to the skin, the scalp can accumulate dead skin cells, product buildup, and toxins, which can hinder hair growth and lead to scalp imbalances. Ayurvedic practices like scalp exfoliation with gentle scrubs made from ingredients like fenugreek, neem, or amla powder can help remove these impurities and promote a healthier scalp environment. Regular scalp detoxification using herbal masks or oils can also revitalize the scalp and stimulate hair follicles.

Diet and Lifestyle Considerations:

Ayurveda recognizes the importance of diet and lifestyle in maintaining healthy hair. Consuming a balanced diet with an emphasis on nutrient-rich foods, such as fresh fruits and vegetables, whole grains, lean proteins, and healthy fats, nourishes the hair follicles from within. Adequate hydration, stress management, and regular exercise also contribute to overall hair health.

Incorporating Ayurvedic principles into your hair and scalp care routine allows you to embrace a natural and holistic approach to hair care. By understanding your dosha and using natural remedies tailored to your hair's needs, you can restore balance, nourish your scalp, and promote healthy, vibrant hair. Remember to be patient, as Ayurvedic hair care focuses on long-term results and the overall well-being of your hair and scalp. With dedication and care, you can unveil the true beauty and strength of your hair through the wisdom of Ayurveda.

Ayurvedic Practices for Maintaining Oral Health: Nurturing Your Smile Naturally

In Ayurveda, oral health is considered essential not only for maintaining a beautiful smile but also for promoting overall well-being. The health of our teeth, gums, and mouth is closely connected to our digestion, immune system, and overall vitality. Ayurvedic principles offer a holistic approach to oral care, focusing on natural remedies, mindful practices, and dietary considerations. By incorporating these practices into our daily routine, we can foster optimal oral health and support the well-being of our entire body. In this article, we explore Ayurvedic practices for maintaining oral health and nurturing a radiant smile.

Oil Pulling (Gandusha):

Oil pulling is a popular Ayurvedic practice for oral health that involves swishing oil in the mouth for several minutes. Traditionally, sesame oil or coconut oil is used for oil pulling, although other oils like sunflower or olive oil can also be used. This practice helps remove toxins, bacteria, and impurities from the mouth, gums, and teeth, promoting oral hygiene. Oil pulling also strengthens the teeth and gums, reduces bad breath, and improves overall oral health.

Herbal Mouth Rinse (Gargle):

Using herbal mouth rinses is an integral part of Ayurvedic oral care. Ayurvedic herbs like neem, clove, triphala, and peppermint are known for their antimicrobial and antiseptic properties. Gargling with herbal mouth rinses helps maintain oral hygiene, freshens the breath, and supports healthy gums. These herbal rinses can be prepared by steeping the herbs in warm water or by using herbal decoctions available in the market.

Tongue Scraping (Jihwa Nirlekhana):

Tongue scraping is a simple yet effective Ayurvedic practice for maintaining oral hygiene. A tongue scraper, usually made of copper or stainless steel, is used to gently scrape the tongue from back to front. This action helps remove accumulated bacteria, toxins, and residue from the surface of the tongue, promoting fresh breath and enhancing overall oral health.

Herbal Tooth Powders and Toothpaste:

Ayurveda offers a range of herbal tooth powders and toothpaste that are free from harsh chemicals commonly found in commercial oral care products. These herbal formulations contain ingredients like neem, clove, cardamom, cinnamon, and licorice, known for their antibacterial and soothing properties. They help maintain healthy gums, prevent tooth decay, and promote fresh breath. Ayurvedic tooth powders can be used by mixing them with water or oil to form a paste, while Ayurvedic toothpaste are available in ready-to-use forms.

Dietary Considerations:

Ayurveda recognizes the connection between oral health and diet. A diet that supports oral health includes foods that are nourishing, easy to digest, and gentle on the teeth and gums. Foods rich in vitamins and minerals, such as fresh fruits and vegetables, whole grains, and lean proteins, help promote strong teeth and healthy gums. Chewing on natural mouth-freshening herbs like fennel seeds or cloves after meals can also aid digestion and freshen the breath.

Mindful Eating and Oral Health:

Practicing mindful eating habits can significantly contribute to oral health. Chewing food thoroughly allows proper mixing of saliva, which contains enzymes important for digestion and the initial breakdown of carbohydrates. Mindful eating also helps avoid overeating, which can burden the digestive system and impact oral health. Additionally, avoiding excessive consumption of sugary and acidic foods and beverages helps prevent tooth decay and gum problems.

Regular Dental Check-ups:

While Ayurvedic practices play a significant role in maintaining oral health, it is important to note that regular dental check-ups are also essential. Professional dental cleanings, examinations, and treatments are vital for detecting and addressing any oral health issues. Integrating Ayurvedic practices with conventional dental care ensures a comprehensive approach to oral health maintenance.

Incorporating Ayurvedic practices into your oral care routine can transform your dental hygiene habits and nurture a vibrant, healthy smile. By embracing natural remedies, mindful practices, and dietary considerations, you can achieve optimal oral health and experience the holistic benefits that Ayurveda offers. So, smile brightly and embrace the wisdom of Ayurveda for radiant and nourished oral well-being.

Ayurvedic Approaches to Aging Gracefully: Embracing the Wisdom of Time

Aging is a natural and inevitable process that we all experience. While we cannot stop the clock, Ayurveda provides a holistic approach to aging gracefully, emphasizing the importance of nurturing our body, mind, and spirit as we journey through the different stages of life. Ayurvedic principles and practices offer valuable insights and techniques to help us embrace the wisdom of time and age with vitality, beauty, and grace. In this article, we explore Ayurvedic approaches to aging gracefully and the key principles that can support us in this transformative journey.

Understanding the Aging Process from an Ayurvedic Perspective:

According to Ayurveda, the aging process is influenced by the balance or imbalance of the three doshas (Vata, Pitta, and Kapha) within our body. As we age, the Vata dosha tends to increase, leading to changes in our physical, mental, and emotional well-being. Understanding our doshic constitution and the imbalances that arise with age helps us tailor our lifestyle, diet, and self-care practices to promote healthy aging.

Balancing Vata Dosha:

Balancing Vata dosha is a key aspect of Ayurvedic approaches to aging gracefully. Vata is associated with qualities of movement, dryness, and lightness. To balance Vata, it is important to maintain a regular daily routine, prioritize self-care practices, and create a nurturing environment. Following a Vata-pacifying diet that includes warm, nourishing foods, healthy fats, and grounding spices helps stabilize Vata and supports healthy aging.

Nourishing the Body:

As we age, it becomes crucial to provide our body with optimal nourishment to maintain vitality and well-being. Ayurveda recommends consuming fresh, nutrient-dense foods that are easy to digest and compatible with our dosha. Including a variety of fruits, vegetables, whole grains, healthy fats, and high-quality proteins in our diet provides essential nutrients, antioxidants, and phytochemicals that support cellular health and combat the effects of aging.

Herbal Support:

Ayurvedic herbs and formulations have been used for centuries to support healthy aging. Herbs like ashwagandha, shatavari, guduchi, and amalaki are known for their rejuvenating properties and their ability to nourish the body and mind. These herbs help strengthen the immune system, enhance vitality, support cognitive function, and promote longevity. Incorporating these herbs into our daily routine can be beneficial in supporting graceful aging.

Daily Self-Care Rituals:

In Ayurveda, daily self-care rituals play a vital role in maintaining overall well-being and supporting healthy aging. Abhyanga, the practice of self-massage with warm oil, helps nourish the skin, improve circulation, and promote relaxation. Regular oil massages not only soothe the body but also calm the mind, reduce stress, and support healthy aging. Additionally, practicing yoga, meditation, and pranayama (breathing exercises) help maintain flexibility, balance, and mental clarity as we age.

Stress Reduction and Emotional Well-being:

Managing stress and nurturing emotional well-being are essential components of aging gracefully. Chronic stress accelerates the aging process and can impact both physical and mental health. Ayurveda emphasizes the importance of stress reduction techniques, such as mindfulness, meditation, and gentle exercise, to cultivate a calm and balanced state of mind. Engaging in activities that bring joy, connecting with loved ones, and cultivating gratitude and positivity contribute to emotional well-being and support healthy aging.

Maintaining a Purposeful Life:

Having a sense of purpose and meaning in life is vital for aging gracefully. Ayurveda encourages us to cultivate our passions, engage in activities that bring fulfillment, and contribute to our community. Nurturing social connections, pursuing hobbies, and continuing to learn and grow throughout our lives keep us engaged, vibrant, and mentally stimulated. A purposeful life adds richness and joy to the aging process.

Embracing the Wisdom of Aging:

Ayurveda teaches us to embrace the wisdom that comes with age and honor the journey of life. As we age, we gain valuable insights, life experiences, and a deeper understanding of ourselves and others. By cultivating self-compassion, self-acceptance, and gratitude for the lessons learned, we can navigate the transitions of aging with grace and wisdom.

In conclusion, Ayurveda offers a holistic and nurturing approach to aging gracefully. By embracing the principles of balancing doshas, nourishing the body, practicing self-care, managing stress, and maintaining a purposeful life, we can navigate the journey of aging with vitality, beauty, and grace. Ayurveda reminds us that aging is a natural and transformative process, and by embracing its wisdom, we can cultivate a life of well-being, fulfillment, and joy at any age.

Ayurveda for Women's Health

- Understanding the unique needs of women's health
- Ayurvedic practices for menstrual health and hormonal balance
- Preconception and pregnancy care in Ayurveda
- Postpartum rejuvenation and self-care practices
- Ayurvedic support for menopause and healthy aging in women

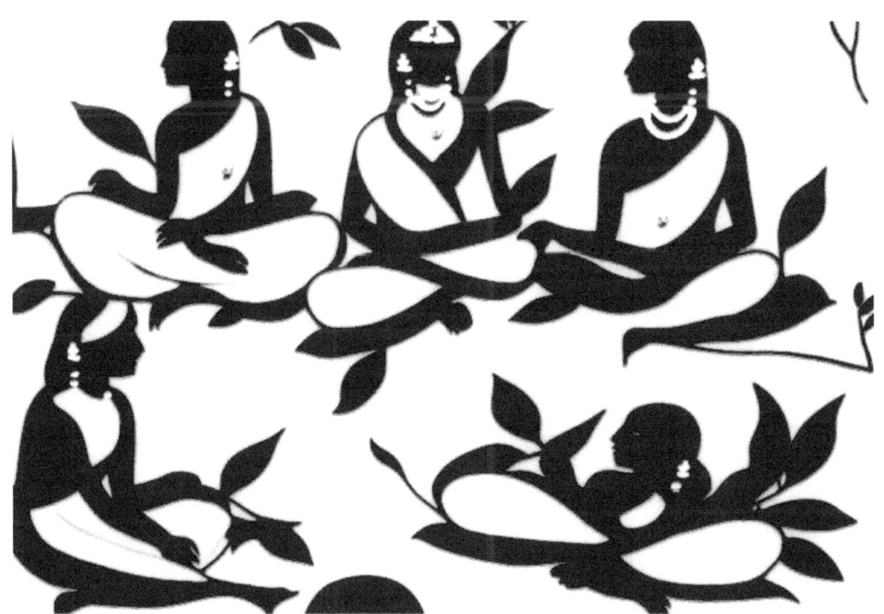

Women's Health

Ayurveda offers profound wisdom and guidance for women's health and well-being. Recognizing that women have unique physical, emotional, and hormonal needs, Ayurveda provides tailored approaches to support women throughout their different life stages, from menstruation to menopause and beyond. With its emphasis on balance, nourishment, and self-care, Ayurveda empowers women to cultivate vibrant health, hormonal harmony, and a deep connection to their innate wisdom and inner radiance. In this article, we delve into the principles and practices of Ayurveda for women's health, exploring how this ancient system can enhance vitality, balance hormones, and nurture overall well-being.

Understanding the Female Body from an Ayurvedic Perspective:

Ayurveda views the female body as a dynamic interplay of energies, influenced by the three doshas: Vata, Pitta, and Kapha. Each woman has a unique constitution, or Prakriti, that determines her inherent qualities and susceptibilities. Ayurveda recognizes the importance of maintaining a balanced state of these doshas for optimal health and well-being. By understanding their individual constitution, women can tailor their lifestyle, diet, and self-care practices to restore balance and support their specific needs.

Honoring the Menstrual Cycle:

Ayurveda celebrates the menstrual cycle as a sacred and vital aspect of a woman's health. It encourages women to honor and listen to their bodies during each phase of their menstrual cycle, adjusting their self-care practices accordingly. Ayurveda offers valuable insights into diet, exercise, rest, and self-care rituals that can help alleviate menstrual discomfort, balance hormones, and promote a harmonious menstrual cycle.

Nourishing the Female Reproductive System:

Ayurveda recognizes the importance of nourishing the female reproductive system to support fertility, hormonal balance, and overall reproductive health. Through specific dietary recommendations, herbal remedies, and lifestyle practices, Ayurveda provides effective tools for maintaining reproductive health and addressing common concerns such as irregular periods, PMS, and fertility challenges.

Pregnancy and Postpartum Care:

Ayurveda places great emphasis on supporting women during pregnancy and the postpartum period. It offers guidelines for proper nutrition, self-care practices, and herbal remedies to nourish the mother and support the healthy development of the baby. Ayurvedic principles also emphasize the importance of postpartum rejuvenation, allowing women to replenish their energy, restore hormonal balance, and bond with their newborn.

Navigating Menopause:

Menopause is a transformative phase in a woman's life, signaling the end of her reproductive years. Ayurveda recognizes the unique challenges that women may face during this transition and provides support for managing symptoms such as hot flashes, mood swings, and hormonal fluctuations. Through Ayurvedic lifestyle adjustments, dietary modifications, herbal remedies, and specific self-care practices, women can navigate menopause with greater ease and embrace the wisdom and freedom that this phase brings.

Self-Care and Emotional Well-being:

Ayurveda encourages women to prioritize self-care and emotional well-being as integral aspects of their overall health. By incorporating practices such as self-massage, meditation, yoga, and stress reduction techniques into their daily routine, women can cultivate a deeper sense of self-love, balance their emotions, and nourish their body, mind, and spirit.

Ayurvedic Practices for Menstrual Health and Hormonal Balance: Nurturing Women's Well-being

Menstruation is a natural and vital process in a woman's life, signaling her reproductive health and vitality. However, many women experience discomfort, irregularities, and hormonal imbalances during their menstrual cycle. Ayurveda, with its holistic approach, offers valuable insights and practices to support menstrual health and hormonal balance. By incorporating Ayurvedic principles into their lifestyle, diet, and self-care routine, women can nurture their well-being and foster a harmonious menstrual cycle. In this article, we explore Ayurvedic practices for menstrual health and hormonal balance.

1. Balanced Diet:

Ayurveda emphasizes the importance of a balanced and nourishing diet to support menstrual health. Foods that are rich in iron, vitamins, minerals, and antioxidants help replenish the body's resources and support healthy blood flow. Incorporating whole grains, fresh fruits and vegetables, legumes, nuts, and seeds into the diet can provide essential nutrients. Ayurveda also recommends avoiding processed foods, caffeine, and excessive sugar, as they may disrupt hormonal balance.

2. Herbal Remedies:

Ayurvedic herbs can be beneficial in supporting menstrual health and hormonal balance. Herbs such as Ashoka, Shatavari, Lodhra, and Aloe Vera have traditionally been used to regulate menstrual cycles, reduce cramps, and support hormonal equilibrium. However, it is important to consult with an Ayurvedic practitioner or healthcare professional before using herbal remedies to ensure they are suitable for individual needs.

3. Stress Reduction:

Stress can have a significant impact on hormonal balance and menstrual health. Ayurveda emphasizes the importance of stress reduction techniques to support overall well-being. Practices such as meditation, deep breathing exercises, yoga, and mindfulness can help reduce stress levels and promote hormonal equilibrium. Taking time for self-care, engaging in activities that bring joy and relaxation, and getting sufficient rest are also crucial for managing stress.

4. Abhyanga (Self-Massage):

Abhyanga, the practice of self-massage with warm oil, is highly valued in Ayurveda for its ability to promote relaxation and balance. Massaging the abdomen and lower back during menstruation can help relieve pain and cramps. Additionally, regular abhyanga throughout the month can support overall hormonal balance and enhance the body's natural healing mechanisms.

5. Yoga and Exercise:

Gentle exercise and yoga can be beneficial for menstrual health and hormonal balance. Practices such as gentle stretching, walking, and specific yoga poses like the Cobra Pose (Bhujangasana) and the Reclining Bound Angle Pose (Supta Baddha Konasana) can help alleviate menstrual discomfort and promote healthy blood flow. However, it is important to listen to the body and avoid strenuous exercise during menstruation.

6. Lifestyle Modifications:

Ayurveda emphasizes the importance of a balanced and disciplined lifestyle for hormonal balance. Following a consistent daily routine (dinacharya) and maintaining regular sleep patterns can support overall well-being and hormone regulation. Creating a calming and nurturing environment at home, establishing healthy sleep habits, and practicing good hygiene during menstruation are also essential for menstrual health.

7. Ayurvedic Treatments:

Ayurveda offers various specialized treatments that can be beneficial for menstrual health and hormonal balance. These treatments, such as Nasya (nasal administration of herbal oils), Panchakarma (detoxification therapies), and herbal steam therapy (Swedana), aim to purify the body, balance the doshas, and promote overall well-being. It is recommended to seek guidance from a qualified Ayurvedic practitioner to determine which treatments are suitable for individual needs.

Thus, Ayurveda provides valuable insights and practices for nurturing menstrual health and achieving hormonal balance. By adopting a holistic approach that includes a balanced diet, herbal remedies, stress reduction techniques, self-care practices, gentle exercise, and lifestyle modifications, women can support their well-being and foster a harmonious menstrual cycle. It is important to remember that every woman is unique, and consulting with an Ayurvedic practitioner can provide personalized guidance and recommendations for achieving optimal menstrual health and hormonal balance.

Preconception and Pregnancy Care in Ayurveda: Nurturing the Journey of Parenthood

The journey of parenthood is a sacred and transformative experience for couples, and Ayurveda offers comprehensive guidance for preconception and pregnancy care. Ayurveda recognizes the significance of preparing the body, mind, and spirit before conception and provides valuable insights into nurturing a healthy pregnancy and supporting the well-being of both the mother and the growing baby. In this article, we explore the principles and practices of preconception and pregnancy care in Ayurveda.

Preconception Care:

Ayurveda emphasizes the importance of preparing the body and optimizing the reproductive health of both parents before conception. This preparation phase, known as Garbhadhana, focuses on balancing the doshas, purifying the body, and promoting vitality. Here are some key aspects of preconception care in Ayurveda:

1. Balancing the Doshas: Balancing the doshas, particularly Vata and Pitta, is essential for promoting fertility and creating an optimal

environment for conception. Ayurvedic lifestyle practices, dietary modifications, and herbal remedies are employed to balance the doshas and promote reproductive health.

2. Detoxification: Ayurveda recommends detoxification therapies, such as Panchakarma, to eliminate toxins from the body and prepare it for pregnancy. These therapies aim to purify the reproductive organs, enhance the quality of reproductive tissues (shukra dhatu), and support overall well-being.

3. Nourishing Diet: Following a nourishing diet is crucial during the preconception phase. Ayurveda emphasizes the consumption of wholesome foods, including fresh fruits, vegetables, whole grains, and healthy fats. It also recommends incorporating specific herbs and spices that support reproductive health, such as Shatavari, Ashwagandha, and Gokshura.

4. Lifestyle Modifications: Adopting a healthy lifestyle is vital for preconception care. This includes managing stress, getting adequate sleep, engaging in regular exercise, and avoiding unhealthy habits such as smoking, excessive alcohol consumption, and recreational drugs.

Pregnancy Care:

Ayurveda offers comprehensive care guidelines throughout the stages of pregnancy, focusing on maintaining the well-being of the mother and supporting the healthy development of the baby. Here are some key aspects of pregnancy care in Ayurveda:

1. Diet and Nutrition: A balanced and nourishing diet is of utmost importance during pregnancy. Ayurveda recommends incorporating foods that are rich in essential nutrients, including fruits, vegetables, whole grains, dairy products, and lean proteins. It also emphasizes the consumption of ghee (clarified butter) for its nourishing and lubricating properties.

2. Prenatal Herbs and Formulas: Ayurveda utilizes specific herbs and herbal formulations to support the health and well-being of the mother and the growing baby during pregnancy. These herbs, such as Shatavari, Ashwagandha, and Brahmi, are chosen based on their nourishing, calming, and rejuvenating properties.

3. Ayurvedic Pregnancy Practices: Ayurveda recommends various practices to promote a healthy and comfortable pregnancy. This includes gentle exercise, prenatal yoga, regular self-massage with Ayurvedic oils, and specific breathing techniques. These practices help improve circulation, reduce stress, and support overall well-being.

4. Emotional Support: Emotional well-being plays a crucial role in a healthy pregnancy. Ayurveda emphasizes the importance of maintaining a positive mindset, practicing relaxation techniques, and nurturing emotional connections with the baby and loved ones.

5. Regular Check-ups: Ayurveda suggests regular prenatal check-ups with a qualified healthcare provider who can monitor the progress of the pregnancy, assess any potential risks, and provide appropriate guidance and support.

6. Postpartum Care: Ayurveda places significant importance on postpartum care, known as Sutika Paricharya. This phase focuses on restoring the mother's strength, nourishing her body, and supporting the bonding between the mother and the baby. It includes specific dietary guidelines, herbal formulations, and postpartum rituals to promote healing and rejuvenation.

Ayurveda provides comprehensive guidance for preconception and pregnancy care, recognizing the importance of preparing the body, mind, and spirit for the journey of parenthood. By embracing Ayurvedic principles, couples can nurture their reproductive health, support a healthy pregnancy, and lay the foundation for the well-being of both the mother and the baby. It is advisable to consult with an experienced Ayurvedic practitioner for personalized guidance and recommendations tailored to individual needs.

Postpartum Rejuvenation and Self-Care Practices: Nurturing the New Mother

The postpartum period is a time of immense transformation and adjustment for new mothers. It is a time to honor and nurture the body, mind, and spirit as they recover from the birthing process and adapt to the demands of caring for a newborn. Ayurveda, with its holistic approach, offers valuable insights and practices to support postpartum rejuvenation and self-care. In this article, we explore the principles and practices of postpartum rejuvenation and self-care according to Ayurveda.

1. Rest and Recovery:

Rest is of utmost importance during the postpartum period. Ayurveda emphasizes the need for ample rest to allow the body to heal and regain strength. New mothers are encouraged to prioritize sleep, take frequent naps, and avoid excessive physical exertion. This restful period supports the restoration of energy and promotes overall well-being.

2. Nutritious Diet:

A nourishing diet is essential for postpartum rejuvenation. Ayurveda recommends consuming warm, cooked, and easily digestible foods that provide nourishment and help restore balance. Including healthy fats, protein-rich foods, whole grains, cooked vegetables, and warming spices can support healing and replenishment. It is advisable to avoid processed and junk foods, excessive caffeine, and spicy or heavy-to-digest foods during this period.

3. Ayurvedic Herbal Remedies:

Ayurvedic herbal remedies can play a vital role in postpartum rejuvenation. Specific herbs and formulations are used to support lactation, enhance digestion, balance hormones, strengthen the uterus, and promote overall well-being. These herbs, such as Shatavari, Ashwagandha, Guduchi, and Triphala, can be consumed under the guidance of an experienced Ayurvedic practitioner.

4. Abhyanga (Self-Massage):

Abhyanga, the practice of self-massage with warm oil, is highly valued in Ayurveda for postpartum rejuvenation. Massaging the body with warm sesame or coconut oil promotes circulation, relieves muscle tension, nourishes the tissues, and enhances relaxation. It is especially beneficial for soothing the joints and supporting the healing of the abdominal area.

5. Warm Baths and Sitz Baths:

Taking warm baths or sitz baths can provide immense comfort and support healing during the postpartum period. Adding herbal infusions, such as chamomile or calendula, to the bathwater can further enhance the healing properties. These baths help relax the body, alleviate muscle soreness, reduce swelling, and promote overall well-being.

6. Belly Binding:

Belly binding is a traditional practice that involves wrapping the abdomen with a cloth or a specially designed postpartum binder. This practice provides support to the abdominal muscles, promotes the contraction of the uterus, and helps in restoring the pre-pregnancy shape of the abdomen. It can be done under the guidance of an experienced professional.

7. Emotional Support:

The postpartum period can bring about a range of emotions for new mothers. Ayurveda recognizes the importance of emotional well-being during this time and emphasizes the need for emotional support. Creating a nurturing and supportive environment, seeking help from loved ones, and engaging in activities that promote relaxation and joy can all contribute to emotional well-being.

8. Gentle Exercise and Yoga:

Gradual re-introduction of gentle exercise and yoga postpartum can be beneficial for rejuvenation. Gentle stretching, pelvic floor exercises, and specific postpartum yoga poses can help improve circulation, tone the muscles, relieve tension, and support overall well-being. It is important to consult with a healthcare professional or a qualified yoga instructor before starting any exercise or yoga routine postpartum.

9. Ayurvedic Postpartum Treatments:

Ayurveda offers specialized postpartum treatments, known as Sutika Chikitsa, that are administered by trained practitioners. These treatments include specific herbal steam therapy, herbal wraps, and oil massages to aid in healing, nourishment, and rejuvenation of the body. These treatments can be customized based on individual needs and are beneficial for overall postpartum recovery.

To sum up, postpartum rejuvenation and self-care are crucial for the well-being of new mothers. Ayurveda provides valuable guidance and practices that promote healing, nourishment, and emotional well-being during this transformative period. By embracing these practices, new mothers can support their recovery, replenish their energy, and foster a deeper connection with themselves and their newborns. It is important to seek guidance from an experienced Ayurvedic practitioner to customize the practices based on individual needs and circumstances.

Ayurvedic Support for Menopause and Healthy Aging in Women: Nurturing the Transition with Balance and Vitality

Menopause is a natural transition that marks the end of a woman's reproductive phase. It is a time of significant physical, emotional, and hormonal changes, and Ayurveda offers valuable support to navigate this transition with grace, balance, and vitality. In this article, we explore the principles and practices of Ayurveda that can help women embrace menopause and promote healthy aging.

Understanding Menopause in Ayurveda:

Ayurveda views menopause as a natural transition in a woman's life and recognizes that each woman experiences it uniquely. According to Ayurveda, the balance of the three doshas, Vata, Pitta, and Kapha, plays a vital role in maintaining well-being during menopause. Understanding one's individual constitution and the changes that occur during this phase can guide the selection of appropriate Ayurvedic practices and remedies.

1. Balancing the Doshas:

During menopause, there is often an increase in Vata dosha, which can lead to symptoms such as dryness, anxiety, and insomnia. Balancing Vata through lifestyle modifications, dietary choices, and herbal remedies can help alleviate these symptoms. Ayurvedic herbs like Ashwagandha, Shatavari, and Brahmi are commonly used to support hormonal balance and promote overall well-being.

2. Nourishing Diet:

A wholesome and nourishing diet is essential during menopause and healthy aging. Ayurveda emphasizes consuming foods that are warm, cooked, and easy to digest. Including a variety of whole grains, fresh fruits and vegetables, healthy fats, and adequate protein supports hormonal balance, bone health, and overall vitality. Herbs and spices such as turmeric, ginger, and cinnamon can be incorporated for their anti-inflammatory and balancing properties.

3. Supporting Bone Health:

Menopause is often associated with a decline in estrogen levels, which can affect bone health. Ayurveda recommends including calcium-rich foods such as sesame seeds, leafy greens, and dairy products to support bone strength. Herbal formulations like Dashamoola and Asthisanhari can also be beneficial for supporting healthy bones and joints.

4. Stress Reduction and Relaxation:

Stress can exacerbate menopausal symptoms, so it is important to prioritize stress reduction techniques and relaxation practices. Ayurveda offers various methods such as daily meditation, deep breathing exercises (pranayama), gentle yoga, and regular self-care rituals to promote relaxation, reduce stress, and support emotional well-being.

5. Ayurvedic Oils and Self-Massage:

Self-massage with Ayurvedic oils, known as Abhyanga, is a nurturing practice that can be especially beneficial during menopause. Massaging the body with warm herbal oils, such as sesame or coconut oil, helps moisturize the skin, improve circulation, alleviate Vata imbalances, and promote overall relaxation and well-being.

6. Supporting Digestive Health:

Ayurveda places great emphasis on maintaining healthy digestion as it is the foundation of overall well-being. During menopause, digestive imbalances may arise. Consuming easily digestible foods, including cooked vegetables, whole grains, and warming spices, can support optimal digestion. Additionally, Ayurvedic herbal formulations like Trikatu and Hingvastak churna can be used to promote healthy digestion.

7. Emotional Well-being:

Menopause can bring about emotional changes and challenges. Ayurveda recognizes the importance of emotional well-being during this phase. Engaging in activities that promote joy, connecting with loved ones, practicing gratitude, and seeking support from a counselor or support group can help navigate the emotional aspects of menopause.

8. Healthy Lifestyle Habits:

Maintaining a healthy lifestyle is key to promoting overall well-being during menopause and healthy aging. Adequate sleep, regular exercise, staying hydrated, and managing stress levels are important lifestyle factors to prioritize. Ayurveda also emphasizes the importance of maintaining a positive mindset, nurturing relationships, and cultivating a sense of purpose and fulfillment in life.

Thus, Ayurveda offers a holistic approach to support women during menopause and promote healthy aging. By embracing Ayurvedic principles, women can nurture their bodies, balance their hormones, and enhance their overall well-being. It is important to consult with an experienced Ayurvedic practitioner for personalized guidance and recommendations based on individual needs and constitution. With Ayurvedic support, women can embrace this transformative phase of life with grace, vitality, and a sense of empowerment.

CHAPTER EIGHT

Ayurveda and Relationships

- The Ayurvedic perspective on relationships
- Nurturing healthy communication and emotional intimacy
- Ayurvedic practices for maintaining harmony in partnerships
- Applying Ayurveda in family and community settings
- Enhancing compassion and connection through Ayurveda

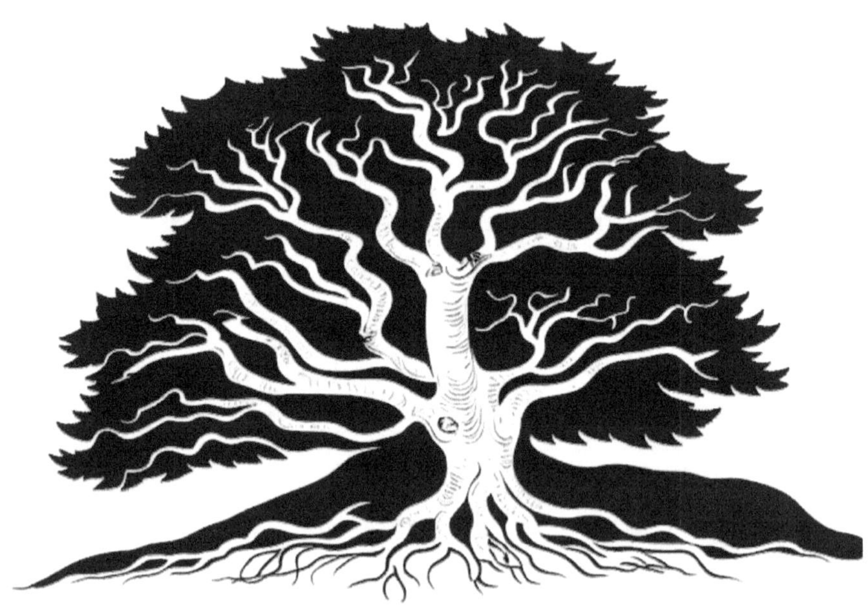

Relationships

Ayurveda offers profound wisdom and insights that can enhance our relationships and foster deeper connection and harmony. In Ayurveda, relationships are seen as an integral part of our overall well-being, recognizing that the quality of our connections significantly impacts our physical, emotional, and spiritual health. By understanding and applying Ayurvedic principles, we can cultivate healthy and fulfilling relationships that nurture and support our growth and well-being. Whether it is our relationship with ourselves, our partners, family members, friends, or colleagues, Ayurveda provides guidance on fostering love, compassion, understanding, and balance in our interactions. In this article, we explore the essence of Ayurveda in the context of relationships and discover how its principles can enhance the way we relate to others and ourselves.

The Ayurvedic perspective on relationships

The Ayurvedic perspective on relationships is deeply rooted in the understanding of the interconnectedness of all beings and the inherent balance and harmony that exists within nature. According to Ayurveda, relationships play a vital role in our overall well-being and are considered a crucial aspect of a healthy and fulfilling life.

In Ayurveda, relationships are viewed as an opportunity for growth, support, and self-realization. It recognizes that each individual has a unique constitution, or dosha, which influences their preferences, behaviors, and tendencies in relationships. Understanding one's dosha and the doshic nature of others can provide valuable insights into how to create balance and harmony in relationships.

Ayurveda emphasizes the importance of cultivating love, compassion, and understanding in all relationships. It encourages open communication, active listening, and empathy as key components of healthy connections. By practicing these qualities, we create a nurturing and supportive environment for both ourselves and our loved ones.

Another essential aspect of Ayurvedic relationships is the concept of "Prakriti" or individual nature. Ayurveda recognizes that each person has unique needs, desires, and ways of expressing love. By understanding and honoring these individual differences, we can foster a deeper sense of connection and acceptance in our relationships.

Furthermore, Ayurveda emphasizes the significance of self-care and self-love in relationships. It teaches that nurturing our own well-being is essential for building healthy and sustainable connections with others. By taking care of our physical, mental, and emotional health, we can show up fully in relationships and contribute to the well-being of those around us.

Ayurveda also acknowledges the influence of the seasons and cycles of life on relationships. Just as nature goes through periods of growth, transformation, and rest, our relationships also experience different phases. Recognizing and embracing these natural rhythms can help us navigate challenges, adapt to changes, and cultivate resilience in our connections.

In summary, the Ayurvedic perspective on relationships revolves around the principles of balance, understanding, and self-care. It encourages us to honor our unique nature and the individuality of others while fostering love, compassion, and open communication. By incorporating Ayurvedic wisdom into our relationships, we can create harmonious and fulfilling connections that support our growth, well-being, and overall happiness.

Ayurvedic Perspective of Nurturing Healthy Communication and Emotional Intimacy: Cultivating Connection and Harmony

In Ayurveda, nurturing healthy communication and emotional intimacy is considered essential for building strong and fulfilling relationships. Ayurveda recognizes that effective communication and emotional intimacy are the pillars of deep connection, understanding, and harmony between individuals. By embracing Ayurvedic principles, we can enhance our ability to express ourselves authentically, listen with empathy, and cultivate emotional intimacy in our relationships.

One of the key aspects of Ayurvedic perspective is the recognition of the unique doshic nature of individuals. Each person has a specific dosha, or mind-body constitution, which influences their communication style and emotional tendencies. Understanding one's dosha can provide valuable insights into how to effectively communicate and foster emotional intimacy with different individuals.

Ayurveda emphasizes the importance of self-awareness and self-reflection in nurturing healthy communication. By cultivating self-awareness, we can better understand our own emotional triggers, communication patterns, and reactions. This awareness allows us to take responsibility for our words and actions, fostering an environment of trust and openness in our relationships.

In Ayurveda, mindful listening is considered a powerful tool for nurturing healthy communication and emotional intimacy. It involves being fully present, paying attention, and empathetically understanding the perspectives and emotions of others. Mindful listening creates space for authentic expression and deepens the connection between individuals.

Ayurveda also recognizes the impact of emotions on communication and intimacy. It teaches that emotions are a natural part of our human experience and should be acknowledged and expressed in a healthy and constructive manner. Suppressed or unexpressed emotions can create barriers to effective communication and hinder the development of emotional intimacy. Ayurveda encourages the cultivation of emotional intelligence, allowing us to understand, process, and express our emotions in a balanced and constructive way.

In addition, Ayurveda emphasizes the importance of creating a nurturing environment for healthy communication and emotional intimacy. This includes practicing self-care, managing stress levels, and creating sacred spaces for open and honest dialogue. Ayurvedic practices such as meditation, yoga, and self-reflection can help individuals cultivate inner balance and clarity, allowing for more authentic and meaningful communication.

Furthermore, Ayurveda highlights the significance of maintaining emotional and energetic balance in relationships. This involves recognizing and respecting the boundaries, needs, and emotions of both oneself and the other person. Creating a safe and non-judgmental space for emotional expression fosters trust and deepens emotional intimacy.

In summary, the Ayurvedic perspective of nurturing healthy communication and emotional intimacy revolves around self-awareness, mindful listening, emotional intelligence, and creating a nurturing environment. By embracing these principles, we can cultivate deep connections, understanding, and harmony in our relationships. Incorporating Ayurvedic practices into our daily lives can enhance our ability to communicate effectively, foster emotional intimacy, and nurture the overall well-being of ourselves and our loved ones.

Ayurvedic Practices for Maintaining Harmony in Partnerships: Nurturing Love and Balance

In Ayurveda, maintaining harmony in partnerships is considered crucial for creating a loving and fulfilling relationship. Ayurvedic principles provide valuable insights and practices that can help couples cultivate balance, understanding, and deep connection. By embracing these practices, couples can nurture their relationship, enhance their bond, and foster a harmonious partnership.

One of the fundamental aspects of Ayurveda is the recognition of individual constitutions or doshas. Each person has a unique mind-body constitution, and understanding these differences can greatly contribute to harmony in partnerships. Ayurveda emphasizes the importance of recognizing and honoring the doshic nature of oneself and one's partner. By understanding each other's preferences, tendencies, and needs, couples can navigate their differences with compassion and respect.

Ayurveda encourages open and authentic communication as a means of maintaining harmony in partnerships. It is essential for couples to create a safe and non-judgmental space where they can express their thoughts, emotions, and needs openly. Effective communication involves active listening, empathy, and a willingness to understand and support each other's perspectives.

Cultivating emotional intimacy is another key aspect of Ayurvedic practices in partnerships. Emotional intimacy involves deep connection, trust, and vulnerability. Ayurveda encourages couples to create rituals of connection, such as regular quality time together, expressing gratitude and appreciation, and engaging in heartfelt conversations. Nurturing emotional intimacy strengthens the bond between partners and enhances overall harmony in the relationship.

Ayurveda emphasizes the importance of shared values and goals in partnerships. Couples can enhance their harmony by aligning their values and working together towards common objectives. This involves discussing and understanding each other's aspirations, dreams, and visions for the future. By supporting each other's growth and working as a team, couples can strengthen their partnership and create a sense of shared purpose.

Maintaining physical intimacy is also considered essential in Ayurveda for fostering harmony in partnerships. Ayurvedic practices emphasize the importance of understanding each other's needs, desires, and rhythms. Ayurveda encourages couples to create a supportive and loving environment where physical intimacy can be nurtured with care, respect, and attention to each other's comfort and pleasure.

Ayurveda recognizes the significance of self-care in maintaining harmony in partnerships. It encourages individuals to prioritize their own well-being, as it directly influences the quality of the relationship. Engaging in self-care practices, such as exercise, meditation, and nurturing routines, helps individuals maintain balance, inner harmony, and a positive mindset, which positively impacts the partnership.

Ayurveda provides valuable practices for maintaining harmony in partnerships. By understanding individual constitutions, practicing open communication, nurturing emotional intimacy, aligning values, maintaining physical intimacy, and prioritizing self-care, couples can create a loving, balanced, and harmonious partnership. Incorporating Ayurvedic principles into daily life strengthens the bond between partners, fosters understanding, and supports the growth and well-being of the relationship.

Applying Ayurveda in Family and Community Settings: Nurturing Wellness and Connection

Ayurveda, the ancient system of holistic living, extends beyond individual well-being and can be applied in family and community settings to foster wellness, harmony, and connection. By embracing Ayurvedic principles and practices together, families and communities can create a supportive environment that promotes health, balance, and overall well-being for all members.

In family settings, Ayurveda encourages the recognition and understanding of each family member's unique constitution or dosha. This understanding helps tailor wellness practices to suit individual needs, ensuring that everyone's well-being is addressed. By considering the doshic influences within the family, such as different food preferences, daily routines, and self-care practices, families can find ways to support each other's health and create a harmonious living environment.

Ayurveda also emphasizes the importance of shared meals and mindful eating in family settings. Eating together as a family promotes a sense of connection, fosters communication, and encourages the appreciation of food and its nourishing qualities. By incorporating Ayurvedic dietary guidelines and considering the tastes and qualities of different ingredients, families can create balanced meals that support optimal health for everyone.

In community settings, Ayurveda can be applied to promote wellness and connection among community members. Community-based wellness initiatives can include workshops or classes on Ayurvedic principles, cooking demonstrations, or group activities that promote physical, mental, and emotional well-being. By sharing knowledge and resources, communities can support each other in implementing Ayurvedic practices and create a sense of collective wellness.

Ayurveda also emphasizes the concept of seva, or selfless service, in community settings. Engaging in acts of service for the well-being of others fosters a sense of connection, empathy, and unity within the community. It can involve volunteering at local organizations, supporting community wellness initiatives, or simply lending a helping hand to those in need. Seva promotes a culture of care and compassion, creating a positive impact on the well-being of both individuals and the community as a whole.

Furthermore, Ayurveda encourages the practice of mindfulness and self-awareness in family and community settings. By cultivating mindfulness, individuals become more present and attentive to their own needs and the needs of others. This awareness can lead to more meaningful interactions, effective communication, and the nurturing of supportive relationships within families and communities.

In summary, applying Ayurveda in family and community settings involves recognizing and honoring individual differences, promoting shared wellness practices, fostering connection through shared meals and activities, engaging in selfless service, and cultivating mindfulness and self-awareness. By incorporating Ayurvedic principles and practices into family and community life, individuals can support each other's well-being, create harmonious living environments, and foster a sense of connection and unity within their families and communities.

Enhancing Compassion and Connection through Ayurveda: Nurturing Empathy and Unity

Ayurveda offers profound insights and practices that can help enhance compassion and connection among individuals and communities. By embracing Ayurvedic principles, we can cultivate empathy, foster deep connections, and promote a sense of unity and well-being in our relationships and interactions.

One of the key aspects of Ayurveda is the recognition of the interconnectedness of all beings. Ayurveda teaches us that we are part of a larger web of life, where our actions and choices have an impact on the well-being of others. This understanding cultivates a sense of compassion, empathy, and interconnectedness, fostering a deeper connection with ourselves, others, and the world around us.

Ayurveda encourages us to practice self-care and self-love as the foundation for enhancing compassion and connection. By prioritizing our own well-being, we cultivate a state of balance, inner harmony, and emotional stability. This enables us to show up fully and authentically in our relationships, being present and available to offer compassion and support to others.

Mindfulness plays a vital role in nurturing compassion and connection through Ayurveda. By cultivating mindfulness, we develop the ability to be fully present and attentive in our interactions. Mindful listening, observing, and responding with empathy allows us to deeply understand and connect with the experiences, emotions, and needs of others. This mindful presence fosters a sense of compassion and creates space for genuine connection and understanding.

Ayurveda emphasizes the importance of fostering positive and loving communication. Choosing our words and tone consciously, speaking with kindness and respect, and actively listening without judgment are essential in enhancing compassion and connection. Ayurveda teaches that the energy and intention behind our words and actions significantly impact the quality of our relationships. By cultivating loving communication, we create an environment that nurtures empathy, trust, and deep connection.

Practicing gratitude is another powerful way to enhance compassion and connection through Ayurveda. By cultivating a grateful mindset, we shift our focus towards acknowledging the blessings and goodness in our lives and in the lives of others. Expressing gratitude, whether through words, acts of kindness, or small gestures, strengthens the bonds of compassion and fosters a sense of unity and connection.

Ayurveda also encourages acts of seva, or selfless service, as a means of enhancing compassion and connection. Engaging in acts of kindness and service without expecting anything in return cultivates a sense of compassion, empathy, and unity with others. Serving those in need, supporting charitable causes, or volunteering in community initiatives not only benefits others but also deepens our own sense of compassion and connection.

Thus, Ayurveda offers powerful tools and practices to enhance compassion and connection in our lives. By prioritizing self-care, cultivating mindfulness, fostering loving communication, practicing gratitude, and engaging in acts of seva, we can nurture empathy, deepen our connections with others, and promote a sense of unity and well-being in our relationships and communities. Through the application of Ayurvedic principles, we can create a more compassionate and connected world, one interaction at a time.

CHAPTER NINE

Ayurveda for the Modern World

- Integrating Ayurveda into a fast-paced lifestyle
- Ayurveda and technology: finding balance in a Digital age
- Ayurvedic approaches to managing chronic diseases
- Ayurvedic perspectives on environmental sustainability
- Cultivating a harmonious and purposeful life

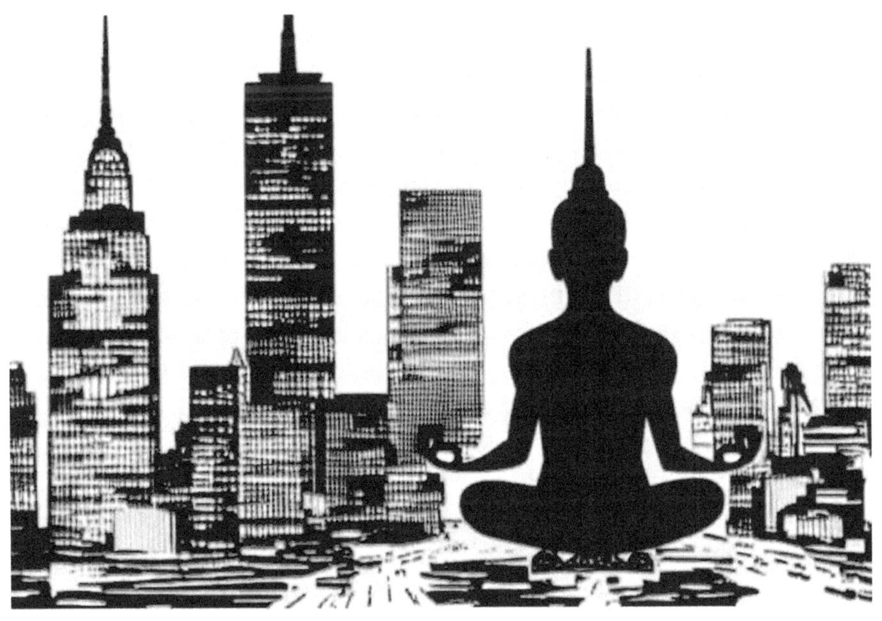

Ayurveda in the Modern World

In today's fast-paced and interconnected world, the need for holistic well-being has never been greater. Amidst the challenges of modern living, Ayurveda, the ancient system of health and balance, offers timeless wisdom and practical guidance to navigate the complexities of our modern lives. Rooted in the belief that true wellness encompasses the mind, body, and spirit, Ayurveda provides a holistic approach to health and emphasizes the importance of individualized care.

Ayurveda acknowledges that each person is unique, with their own constitution and specific needs. It recognizes that what works for one person may not work for another. This personalized approach to wellness is particularly relevant in the modern world, where the one-size-fits-all approach often falls short. Ayurveda offers a tailored approach to well-being, empowering individuals to embrace their unique qualities and make conscious choices that support their overall health and balance.

Beyond symptom management, Ayurveda seeks to address the root cause of imbalance, viewing health as an intricate interplay of physical, mental, emotional, and spiritual factors. It emphasizes the importance of lifestyle practices, such as mindful eating, self-care rituals, and daily routines, as key pillars of well-being. By adopting Ayurvedic principles and practices, individuals can cultivate a deeper sense of connection to themselves, others, and the natural world around them.

In the modern world, where stress, chronic diseases, and lifestyle imbalances are prevalent, Ayurveda offers a refreshing perspective on prevention and holistic healing. It recognizes that true wellness extends beyond the absence of disease and strives to bring individuals into a state of optimal health and balance. By embracing Ayurvedic practices such as mindful eating, meditation, yoga, and herbal remedies, individuals can proactively support their well-being and cultivate a sense of harmony in their lives.

Moreover, Ayurveda invites us to reconnect with nature and live in harmony with the rhythms and cycles of the natural world. In a time when technology and urbanization have disconnected us from the natural environment, Ayurveda reminds us of our inherent connection to the Earth and the healing power of natural elements. By incorporating Ayurvedic principles into our lives, we can reclaim a sense of balance, rootedness, and reverence for the natural world.

Integrating Ayurveda into a Fast-Paced Lifestyle: Nurturing Balance and Well-Being

In the midst of our fast-paced and demanding modern lifestyles, finding balance and maintaining well-being can often feel like a daunting task. However, Ayurveda, the ancient system of health and harmony, offers valuable insights and practical approaches to help us integrate its principles into our busy lives. By embracing Ayurveda, we can foster balance, nurture our well-being, and navigate the challenges of a fast-paced lifestyle with grace and mindfulness.

One of the fundamental principles of Ayurveda is the recognition of individual uniqueness. Each person has a distinct constitution, known as dosha, which influences their physical and mental characteristics. By understanding our dosha, we can tailor our lifestyle choices, including diet, exercise, and daily routines, to support our specific needs. This personalized approach allows us to optimize our energy, manage stress, and maintain balance amidst a hectic lifestyle.

Mindful Eating: In a fast-paced lifestyle, it is common to eat on the go or resort to quick, unhealthy food choices. However, Ayurveda emphasizes the importance of mindful eating. Taking time to sit down, savor each bite, and pay attention to the tastes and textures of our food allows us to better digest and assimilate nutrients. Incorporating Ayurvedic dietary guidelines, such as favoring fresh, whole foods and avoiding processed and heavy foods, can support optimal digestion and nourishment.

Daily Routine: Establishing a daily routine, known as dinacharya, is key to maintaining balance and grounding amidst a busy lifestyle. Ayurveda suggests incorporating self-care practices, such as tongue scraping, oil pulling, and self-massage (abhyanga), into our morning routine to promote detoxification, improve circulation, and nurture the body. Setting aside time for relaxation, meditation, or gentle yoga in the evening can help release accumulated stress and prepare the mind for restful sleep.

Managing Stress: Stress is a common challenge in a fast-paced lifestyle, but Ayurveda offers effective tools for managing it. Incorporating stress-reducing practices, such as pranayama (breathing exercises), meditation, and mindfulness, can help cultivate a sense of calm and balance. Additionally, Ayurvedic herbs and adaptogens, such as ashwagandha and brahmi, can support the body's resilience to stress and promote overall well-being.

Simplifying and Prioritizing: Ayurveda teaches us the importance of simplifying our lives and prioritizing what truly matters. In a fast-paced lifestyle, we may find ourselves overwhelmed with commitments and responsibilities. By identifying our priorities and simplifying our schedules, we can create space for self-care, relaxation, and meaningful connections. Learning to say no, setting boundaries, and delegating tasks when possible are valuable strategies for nurturing balance and well-being.

Connecting with Nature: Despite our fast-paced lives, it is crucial to reconnect with nature regularly. Spending time in nature, even if it's a short walk in a park or tending to a small garden, can have profound benefits for our overall well-being. Ayurveda recognizes the healing power of nature and encourages us to align with the natural rhythms and cycles. Taking breaks outdoors, practicing earthing (walking barefoot on natural surfaces), and incorporating elements of nature into our living spaces can help foster a sense of grounding and harmony.

Seeking Support: Integrating Ayurveda into a fast-paced lifestyle can be challenging, but seeking support from Ayurvedic practitioners, wellness coaches, or joining Ayurvedic communities can provide guidance and encouragement. These resources can help us navigate the intricacies of Ayurvedic principles and offer practical suggestions tailored to our specific needs and lifestyle.

In summary, integrating Ayurveda into a fast-paced lifestyle is about finding harmony amidst the busyness and prioritizing self-care and well-being. By embracing Ayurvedic principles such as mindful eating, establishing a daily routine, managing stress, simplifying our lives, connecting with nature, and seeking support, we can nurture balance, enhance our overall well-being, and thrive in the midst of a fast-paced world. Ayurveda reminds us to slow down, listen to our bodies, and make conscious choices that support our health and happiness.

Ayurveda and Technology: Finding Balance in a Digital Age

In today's digital age, technology has become an integral part of our daily lives. While it brings numerous benefits and conveniences, it also poses challenges to our overall well-being and balance. Ayurveda, the ancient system of health and harmony, offers valuable insights and practices to help us navigate the impact of technology and find a healthy balance in our relationship with it.

Ayurveda recognizes that everything in the universe, including technology, is composed of the five elements (earth, water, fire, air, and space) and has the potential to influence our doshas (unique mind-body constitution). Technology, with its fast-paced nature and constant stimulation, can exacerbate the vata dosha, which is associated with movement, change, and overstimulation. Excessive use of technology can lead to imbalances such as restlessness, anxiety, sleep disturbances, and decreased focus.

Here are some Ayurvedic practices and principles that can help us maintain balance in the digital age:

1. Establish Boundaries: Set boundaries around technology use to prevent excessive screen time and overstimulation. Designate tech-free zones or periods in your day, such as during meals, before bedtime, or in the first hour after waking up. This allows for dedicated time for self-care, relaxation, and connection with yourself and others.

2. Practice Mindful Technology Use: Approach technology with mindfulness and awareness. Before engaging with your devices, take a moment to check in with yourself. Ask yourself if you genuinely need to use technology at that moment or if there are other nourishing activities you can engage in instead. Be conscious of how technology makes you feel and its impact on your mental and emotional well-being.

3. Digital Detoxes: Consider periodically taking breaks from technology, such as a digital detox weekend or unplugging for a few hours each day. Use this time to engage in activities that promote relaxation, creativity, and connection with nature and loved ones. Disconnecting from technology allows for rejuvenation and helps restore balance.

4. Mind-Body Practices: Incorporate mind-body practices, such as yoga, meditation, and pranayama (breathing exercises), into your daily routine. These practices help calm the mind, reduce stress, and promote inner balance. Engaging in these practices can counterbalance the overstimulation and mental restlessness that technology can induce.

5. Outdoor Time: Spend time in nature regularly to counterbalance the indoor and sedentary nature of technology use. Nature has a grounding and calming effect on the mind and body. Take walks, engage in outdoor activities, or simply sit in a natural setting to reconnect with the elements and find solace away from screens.

6. Ayurvedic Self-Care: Prioritize self-care practices that help balance the effects of technology. This may include abhyanga (self-massage) with

warm oil to calm the nervous system, practicing neti (nasal cleansing) to support respiratory health, or incorporating calming herbs like ashwagandha or brahmi into your routine to nourish the nervous system.

7. Conscious Media Consumption: Be discerning about the content you consume through technology. Choose media that uplifts, educates, and inspires you rather than feeds into negative emotions or drains your energy. Seek a balance between entertainment and nourishing information.

8. Cultivate Real-Life Connections: While technology provides opportunities for virtual connections, prioritize building and nurturing real-life relationships. Engage in face-to-face interactions, spend quality time with loved ones, and cultivate meaningful connections that promote emotional well-being.

Remember that technology itself is not inherently negative; it is the way we engage with it that determines its impact on our well-being. Ayurveda encourages us to find a balance that supports our physical, mental, and emotional health. By incorporating these Ayurvedic practices and principles, we can navigate the digital age with mindfulness, intention, and an emphasis on well-being, finding harmony between the benefits of technology and our overall balance and happiness.

Ayurvedic Approaches to Managing Chronic Diseases in the Modern World

Chronic diseases have become increasingly prevalent in the modern world, and managing them requires a comprehensive and holistic approach. Ayurveda, the ancient system of health and harmony, offers valuable insights and practices that can support the management of chronic diseases. By addressing the root causes, nurturing balance, and promoting overall well-being, Ayurveda provides a multifaceted approach to managing chronic conditions.

1. Individualized Approach: Ayurveda recognizes that each person is unique, and chronic diseases manifest differently in different individuals. Therefore, an individualized approach is essential in Ayurvedic management. Ayurvedic practitioners consider an individual's dosha (mind-body constitution), prakriti (natural state), vikruti (current state), and specific imbalances. This personalized approach allows for tailored treatment plans that address the specific needs of each individual.

2. Balancing the Doshas: Ayurveda emphasizes the balance of the three doshas (Vata, Pitta, and Kapha) as a foundation for health. Imbalances in the doshas contribute to the development and progression of chronic diseases. Ayurvedic treatments focus on restoring balance through dietary modifications, herbal remedies, lifestyle adjustments, and specific therapies that address the imbalances in the doshas.

3. Mind-Body Connection: Ayurveda recognizes the intimate connection between the mind and body in the manifestation and management of chronic diseases. Stress, emotional imbalances, and negative thought patterns can exacerbate chronic conditions. Ayurvedic practices such as meditation, pranayama (breathing exercises), and yoga help calm the mind, reduce stress, and promote emotional well-being. Addressing the mind-body connection is an integral part of managing chronic diseases.

4. Diet and Nutrition: Ayurvedic nutrition plays a crucial role in managing chronic diseases. Ayurveda emphasizes a whole-foods, plant-based diet that is tailored to the individual's dosha and the specific needs of the condition. Dietary recommendations may include incorporating fresh fruits and vegetables, whole grains, legumes, healthy fats, and spices with medicinal properties. Avoiding processed foods, excessive sugar, and unhealthy fats is also emphasized.

5. Herbal Remedies: Ayurvedic herbal remedies have been used for centuries to support the management of chronic diseases. Herbs such as turmeric, ashwagandha, triphala, guggul, and tulsi have potent anti-inflammatory, antioxidant, and immune-modulating properties. Ayurvedic practitioners prescribe herbs based on the individual's constitution and the specific needs of the condition, aiming to address the underlying imbalances and support overall well-being.

6. Panchakarma: Panchakarma is a renowned Ayurvedic detoxification and rejuvenation therapy. It is particularly beneficial in chronic diseases as it helps remove accumulated toxins, restore balance, and strengthen the body's natural healing abilities. Panchakarma treatments typically include specialized massage, herbal steam therapy, enemas, and nasal therapies. The treatments are tailored to the individual's needs and are performed under the guidance of trained Ayurvedic practitioners.

7. Lifestyle Modifications: Ayurveda recognizes the importance of lifestyle in managing chronic diseases. Adopting healthy lifestyle habits such as regular exercise, adequate sleep, stress management techniques, and maintaining a consistent daily routine can significantly contribute to

managing chronic conditions. Ayurvedic practitioners provide guidance on lifestyle modifications that support overall well-being and balance.

8. Integrative Approach: Ayurveda can complement conventional medical treatments for chronic diseases. It is important to work with a knowledgeable healthcare provider who can integrate Ayurvedic principles and practices into an individual's overall treatment plan. Collaborating with healthcare professionals from various disciplines ensures a holistic approach to managing chronic diseases.

Ayurveda encourages individuals to take an active role in managing their health and well-being. It emphasizes self-care, self-awareness, and lifestyle modifications that nurture balance and support the body's innate healing capabilities. By incorporating Ayurvedic principles and practices into the management of chronic diseases, individuals can experience improved quality of life, enhanced well-being, and better overall health outcomes.

Ayurvedic Perspectives on Environmental Sustainability: Nurturing Harmony with Nature

Ayurveda, the ancient Indian system of medicine and holistic living, recognizes the intrinsic connection between human well-being and the health of the environment. It emphasizes the importance of living in harmony with nature and offers valuable perspectives and practices for promoting environmental sustainability. Ayurveda acknowledges that a healthy environment is essential for the well-being of individuals, communities, and the planet as a whole. Here, we delve into the Ayurvedic perspectives on environmental sustainability and the practices that can help us nurture balance and harmony with our natural surroundings.

1. Interconnectedness: Ayurveda views everything in the universe as interconnected and interdependent. It recognizes that human beings are an integral part of nature and that our well-being is intimately linked to the health of the environment. Ayurveda teaches us to cultivate a deep respect and reverence for nature, acknowledging that our actions have a direct impact on the ecosystem.

2. Elemental Balance: Ayurveda understands the world in terms of the five elements: earth, water, fire, air, and space. It recognizes that these elements exist not only within us but also in the environment. Ayurveda teaches us to strive for balance and harmony in our relationship with the elements, avoiding overconsumption and waste. By aligning our actions

with the natural elements, we contribute to the sustainability of the environment.

3. Sustainable Agriculture: Ayurveda promotes the cultivation and consumption of organic, locally sourced, and seasonal foods. It encourages sustainable agricultural practices that minimize the use of synthetic chemicals and support the natural fertility of the soil. Ayurvedic principles guide us to make mindful choices about the food we consume, considering its impact on our health and the environment.

4. Conservation of Natural Resources: Ayurveda emphasizes the responsible use and conservation of natural resources such as water, air, and forests. It encourages us to use these resources judiciously and minimize waste. We should encourage practices such as rainwater harvesting, tree planting, and energy conservation to contribute to the sustainable management of resources.

5. Mindful Waste Management: Emphasize the importance of proper waste management to prevent pollution and protect the environment. It encourages recycling, composting, and reducing the use of non-biodegradable materials. By practicing mindful waste management, we contribute to a cleaner and healthier environment for ourselves and future generations.

6. Eco-friendly Lifestyle: Ayurveda advocates for an eco-friendly lifestyle that embraces simplicity, minimalism, and conscious consumption. It encourages us to reduce our ecological footprint by making conscious choices about the products we use, opting for sustainable and natural alternatives whenever possible. Ayurveda teaches us to live in harmony with nature rather than exploiting it for our own gain.

7. Connection with Nature: Ayurveda recognizes the healing power of nature and the importance of spending time in natural surroundings. It encourages us to reconnect with the natural world through activities such as walking in nature, gardening, and practicing yoga outdoors. This connection with nature not only enhances our well-being but also deepens our appreciation for the environment and inspires us to protect and preserve it. Ayurveda is a great teacher of seeing ourselves in everything around us including trees, insects, mountains, rivers, and so on.

8. Advocacy and Education: Ayurveda encourages individuals to become advocates for environmental sustainability and share their knowledge with others. By educating ourselves and raising awareness about the importance of sustainable living, we can inspire positive change in our communities and

beyond.

Incorporating Ayurvedic perspectives on environmental sustainability into our lives is a way to align our actions with the principles of balance, interconnectedness, and reverence for nature. By nurturing the health of the environment, we simultaneously nurture our own well-being and contribute to a more sustainable future for generations to come. Let us embrace these principles and make conscious choices that support environmental sustainability in all aspects of our lives.

Ayurvedic Perspectives of Cultivating a Harmonious and Purposeful Life: Establishing Balance, Purpose, and Well-Being

Ayurveda, the ancient Indian system of medicine and holistic living, offers profound insights and practices for cultivating a harmonious and purposeful life. It recognizes that true well-being and fulfillment arise from aligning our actions, thoughts, and intentions with our unique purpose and the rhythms of nature. Ayurveda provides a holistic framework that encompasses physical, mental, emotional, and spiritual aspects of life, guiding us towards balance, inner harmony, and a sense of purpose. Here, we delve into the Ayurvedic perspectives on cultivating a harmonious and purposeful life and the practices that can support us on this transformative journey.

1. Self-Discovery and Self-Awareness: Ayurveda emphasizes self-discovery and self-awareness as fundamental pillars of cultivating a purposeful life. Through self-reflection, introspection, and mindful observation of our thoughts, emotions, and behaviors, we gain insight into our true nature, desires, strengths, and areas for growth. Ayurveda encourages us to cultivate a deep understanding of ourselves, allowing us to align our actions and choices with our authentic selves and purpose.

2. Living in Harmony with Nature: Ayurveda recognizes that we are intimately connected to the natural world and its rhythms. By aligning our lifestyle, routines, and choices with the cycles of nature, we create a harmonious and supportive environment for growth and well-being. This includes observing daily and seasonal rhythms, incorporating natural elements into our living spaces, and spending time in nature to nurture a sense of connection and reverence for the world around us.

3. Ayurvedic Daily Routine (Dinacharya): The Ayurvedic daily routine, known as Dinacharya, provides a framework for structuring our days in

a balanced and purposeful manner. It includes practices such as waking up early, self-care rituals (like tongue scraping and oil pulling), meditation or mindfulness, exercise or yoga, nourishing meals, and a regular sleep schedule. Following a consistent daily routine helps establish a sense of stability, rhythm, and intention in our lives.

4. Mind-Body-Spirit Integration: Ayurveda recognizes the interconnectedness of the mind, body, and spirit in cultivating a harmonious and purposeful life. It emphasizes the importance of nurturing all aspects of our being through practices that promote physical health, mental clarity, emotional balance, and spiritual growth. This may include adopting a nourishing diet, engaging in regular exercise or yoga, practicing mindfulness and meditation, cultivating positive relationships, and engaging in self-reflection or spiritual practices that resonate with us.

5. Cultivating Sattva: Ayurveda acknowledges the three Gunas (qualities of nature) - Sattva (purity), Rajas (activity), and Tamas (inertia). Cultivating Sattva, the quality of purity, clarity, and harmony, is considered essential for living a purposeful life. Sattvic practices include consuming pure, whole foods; engaging in uplifting activities; fostering positive relationships; and cultivating qualities such as compassion, love, gratitude, and forgiveness. By aligning our actions with Sattva, we create a conducive environment for personal growth and the realization of our purpose.

6. Pursuing Dharma: Ayurveda recognizes the significance of living in alignment with our dharma, our unique purpose or calling in life. Discovering and pursuing our dharma involves aligning our passions, talents, values, and actions with a greater sense of meaning and service. Ayurveda teaches us to listen to our inner voice, follow our heart's desires, and make choices that are in harmony with our purpose, allowing us to experience a deep sense of fulfillment and contribute meaningfully to the world.

7. Cultivating Mindfulness and Gratitude: Ayurveda emphasizes the practice of mindfulness and gratitude as powerful tools for cultivating a harmonious and purposeful life. By bringing our awareness to the present moment, we can fully engage in our experiences, make conscious choices, and appreciate the beauty and abundance that surrounds us. Expressing gratitude for the blessings in our lives helps shift our focus towards positivity, contentment, and a deeper sense of fulfillment.

8. Seeking Support and Connection: Ayurveda recognizes the importance of seeking support and connection in our journey towards a

harmonious and purposeful life. This may involve seeking guidance from Ayurvedic practitioners, mentors, or wise teachers, as well as nurturing supportive relationships with family, friends, and community. Building a network of like-minded individuals who share our values and aspirations provides encouragement, inspiration, and accountability on our path.

By embracing the Ayurvedic perspectives on cultivating a harmonious and purposeful life and incorporating the practices that resonate with us, we can embark on a transformative journey towards balance, well-being, and fulfillment. As we deepen our self-awareness, align with our purpose, and live in harmony with nature and our inner truth, we create the conditions for a truly meaningful and purposeful life. Let us embrace these teachings, honor our unique journey, and create a life that is rich in meaning, joy, and connection.

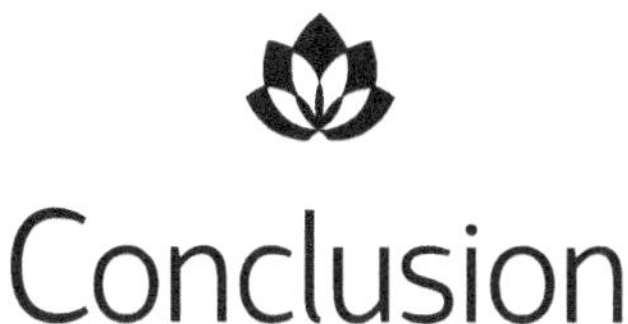

CHAPTER TEN

Conclusion

- Embracing Ayurveda as a lifelong journey
- The transformative power of Ayurveda in everyday life
- Practical tips for incorporating Ayurvedic wisdom

Embracing Ayurveda as a Lifelong Journey: For Us and For Generations to Come

Ayurveda, the ancient Indian system of medicine and holistic living, is not just a quick fix or a temporary solution. It is a profound philosophy and way of life that offers a lifelong journey of self-discovery, well-being, and balance. Embracing Ayurveda is an ongoing process that involves integrating its principles into every aspect of your life, cultivating self-awareness, and nurturing a deep connection with yourself and the world around you. Here, we delve into the essence of embracing Ayurveda as a lifelong journey and the transformative aspects it brings to our lives.

1. The Power of Self-Discovery: Ayurveda invites us to embark on a journey of self-discovery, exploring our unique mind-body constitution (dosha) and understanding our individual needs and tendencies. By gaining self-awareness and recognizing the patterns and imbalances within us, we can make informed choices that promote well-being and cultivate a deep connection with ourselves.

2. Adapting to Life's Seasons: Just as nature goes through different seasons, our lives also go through phases of change and transformation. Ayurveda teaches us to adapt to these seasons of life, recognizing that our needs may shift and evolve. By embracing Ayurveda as a lifelong journey, we learn to navigate these changes with grace, adjusting our diet, lifestyle,

and practices to maintain balance and harmony.

3. Continuous Learning and Growth: Ayurveda is a vast and profound system of knowledge that offers a lifetime of learning and growth. As we deepen our understanding of Ayurvedic principles, we uncover new insights and discover how to apply them in our daily lives. Embracing Ayurveda as a lifelong journey means being open to continuous learning, exploring new perspectives, and expanding our understanding of ourselves and the world.

4. Integration into Everyday Life: Ayurveda is not a separate entity from our daily lives; it is meant to be integrated into every aspect of our existence. Embracing Ayurveda involves incorporating its principles into our routines, choices, and interactions. Whether it's mindful eating, self-care rituals, or conscious relationships, Ayurveda becomes a guiding force in our everyday actions, supporting our well-being and fostering a sense of harmony.

5. Cultivating Balance and Well-being: Ayurveda's primary goal is to establish and maintain balance within our bodies, minds, and spirits. Embracing Ayurveda as a lifelong journey means continually seeking balance and adjusting our lifestyle and practices to restore harmony when imbalances arise. By nurturing balance, we enhance our overall well-being and create a solid foundation for a fulfilling life.

6. Honoring the Mind-Body-Spirit Connection: Ayurveda recognizes the profound interplay between the mind, body, and spirit. Embracing Ayurveda involves acknowledging and honoring this connection, treating each aspect with equal importance. By cultivating practices that nourish our physical, mental, and spiritual well-being, we embark on a transformative journey that promotes holistic health and inner harmony.

7. Self-Care as a Priority: Ayurveda places great emphasis on self-care as a means of nurturing well-being and balance. Embracing Ayurveda involves prioritizing self-care rituals, such as Abhyanga (self-massage), meditation, yoga, and self-reflection. By dedicating time and attention to our own needs, we replenish our energy, cultivate self-love, and create a solid foundation for a lifelong journey of well-being.

8. Connection with Nature and the Universe: Ayurveda teaches us that we are intimately connected to the natural world and the universe as a whole. Embracing Ayurveda involves fostering a deep connection with nature, aligning our lifestyle and choices with the rhythms and cycles of the Earth. By spending time in nature, practicing gratitude, and embracing

the interconnectedness of all things, we nourish our souls and experience a sense of purpose and belonging.

9. Embracing the Present Moment: Ayurveda encourages us to embrace the present moment fully. By cultivating mindfulness and being fully present in each experience, we deepen our connection with ourselves and the world around us. This presence allows us to make conscious choices, savor the beauty of each moment, and cultivate a sense of purpose and fulfillment in our lives.

10. Evolving Relationship with Ayurveda: Embracing Ayurveda as a lifelong journey means developing a dynamic and evolving relationship with this ancient wisdom. As we navigate through different stages of life, our understanding and application of Ayurvedic principles may change. Embracing Ayurveda as a lifelong journey involves adapting and evolving our practices to meet our ever-changing needs while staying rooted in the core principles of balance, well-being, and self-discovery.

In a nutshell, embracing Ayurveda as a lifelong journey is an invitation to embark on a transformative path of self-discovery, well-being, and balance. By integrating Ayurvedic principles into our daily lives, cultivating self-awareness, and nurturing a deep connection with ourselves and the world, we embark on a journey that enriches every aspect of our existence. Embrace Ayurveda as a lifelong companion and allow it to guide you towards a harmonious, purposeful, and fulfilling life.

The Transformative Power of Ayurveda in Everyday Life: For A Complete Life

Ayurveda offers a transformative approach to life that goes beyond mere physical health. Rooted in the belief that balance is the key to well-being, Ayurveda empowers individuals to make conscious choices and cultivate a harmonious relationship with themselves, others, and the world around them. By embracing Ayurveda in everyday life, one can unlock the transformative power of this ancient wisdom and experience profound shifts in physical, mental, and spiritual well-being. Here, we explore the various ways Ayurveda can positively impact and transform our everyday lives.

1. Mind-Body Awareness: Ayurveda emphasizes the importance of self-awareness and understanding the unique constitution of our mind and body. Through Ayurveda, we learn to recognize our doshas (Vata, Pitta, and

Kapha) and understand how they influence our physical and mental well-being. This awareness enables us to make informed choices about our diet, lifestyle, and daily routines that support balance and prevent imbalances or health issues from arising.

2. Personalized Approach to Health: Ayurveda recognizes that each individual is unique and requires a personalized approach to health. By understanding our constitution and recognizing our unique needs, we can tailor our diet, lifestyle, and self-care practices to suit our specific requirements. This personalized approach fosters a deep sense of self-care and empowers us to take charge of our own health and well-being.

3. Balance in Diet and Nutrition: Ayurveda places great emphasis on the role of food in maintaining balance and promoting health. By following Ayurvedic principles of diet and nutrition, we can make conscious choices about the foods we consume and their impact on our well-being. Ayurveda categorizes foods based on their taste (rasa), heating or cooling properties (virya), and post-digestive effect (vipaka) to guide us in selecting a balanced and nourishing diet.

4. Holistic Lifestyle Practices: Ayurveda advocates for the integration of holistic lifestyle practices that support overall well-being. These practices include daily routines (dinacharya), self-care rituals (dinacharya), yoga, meditation, and mindfulness. By incorporating these practices into our daily lives, we create a foundation for balance, vitality, and spiritual growth.

5. Embracing Nature's Rhythms: Ayurveda recognizes the interconnectedness between human beings and nature. By aligning ourselves with the rhythms of nature, such as the cycles of the day, the seasons, and the lunar calendar, we can harmonize our internal and external environments. This connection to nature helps us find balance and attune to the natural flow of life.

6. Emotional and Mental Well-being: Ayurveda acknowledges the profound influence of emotions and mental states on our overall well-being. By adopting Ayurvedic practices like meditation, pranayama (breathing exercises), and self-reflection, we can cultivate emotional balance, reduce stress, and enhance mental clarity. Ayurvedic herbs and therapies also offer support for emotional well-being, helping to alleviate conditions like anxiety and depression.

7. Sustainable and Ethical Choices: Ayurveda encourages us to make conscious choices that not only benefit our individual health but also contribute to the well-being of the planet and its inhabitants. By embracing

sustainable and ethical practices in our daily lives, such as choosing organic and locally sourced foods, using natural and eco-friendly products, and respecting the environment, we become active participants in creating a healthier and more sustainable world.

8. Cultivating Spiritual Awareness: Ayurveda recognizes the spiritual aspect of human existence and encourages the cultivation of spiritual awareness. Through practices like meditation, self-reflection, and

the pursuit of self-realization, Ayurveda provides a pathway to connect with our inner selves and tap into our innate wisdom and higher consciousness. This spiritual dimension adds depth and meaning to our everyday lives, transforming our perspective and opening doors to profound personal growth and transformation.

Thus, Ayurveda offers a transformative framework for living a balanced, healthy, and purposeful life. By integrating Ayurvedic principles and practices into our everyday lives, we can nurture balance, health, and well-being on all levels – physical, mental, emotional, and spiritual. The transformative power of Ayurveda lies in its holistic approach, personalized care, and deep connection to nature and the self. Embrace Ayurveda as a lifelong journey, and experience the profound transformation it can bring to your everyday life.

Practical Tips for Incorporating Ayurvedic Wisdom into Everyday Life

Ayurveda is a wealth of wisdom and practices that can enhance our well-being and bring balance to our lives. By incorporating Ayurvedic principles into our daily routines and choices, we can experience profound shifts in our physical, mental, and emotional health. Here are some practical tips for incorporating Ayurvedic wisdom into your everyday life:

1. Discover Your Ayurvedic Constitution: Understanding your unique Ayurvedic constitution, or dosha, is key to making informed choices. Take an online dosha quiz or consult with an Ayurvedic practitioner to determine your dominant dosha (Vata, Pitta, or Kapha) and understand your individual needs.

2. Align with the Rhythms of Nature: Ayurveda emphasizes living in harmony with nature's rhythms. Wake up early in the morning when the air is fresh, and establish a daily routine that aligns with the natural cycles of the day. This includes eating meals at regular times and winding down in

the evening to prepare for a restful sleep.

3. Mindful Eating: Pay attention to what and how you eat. Chew your food thoroughly, savor each bite, and eat in a calm and relaxed environment. Focus on incorporating fresh, seasonal, and organic foods into your diet. Emphasize whole grains, fruits, vegetables, legumes, and healthy fats while reducing processed foods, artificial additives, and refined sugars.

4. Digestive Health: Ayurveda places great importance on a healthy digestive system. Practice mindful eating, and allow time for proper digestion between meals. Consider incorporating spices like ginger, cumin, coriander, and fennel, which can aid digestion. Avoid overeating and eating heavy meals late at night.

5. Daily Self-Care Rituals: Establish daily self-care rituals to nourish your body, mind, and spirit. This may include practices like self-massage (abhyanga) with warm oil, tongue scraping, oil pulling, and gentle exercise or yoga. These rituals promote relaxation, improve circulation, and support overall well-being.

6. Stress Management: Ayurveda recognizes the impact of stress on our health. Incorporate stress management techniques into your daily routine, such as meditation, deep breathing exercises, yoga, or engaging in activities that bring you joy and relaxation. Prioritize self-care and create space for relaxation and rejuvenation.

7. Herbal Support: Explore the healing properties of Ayurvedic herbs. Consult with an Ayurvedic practitioner to identify herbs and herbal formulas that can support your specific needs. Herbs like ashwagandha, turmeric, brahmi, and triphala are known for their balancing and rejuvenating properties.

8. Create a Harmonious Environment: Surround yourself with a nurturing and harmonious environment. Declutter your living spaces, bring in natural elements like plants and fresh air, and create a peaceful ambiance through soft lighting and soothing scents. Consider incorporating Ayurvedic principles of Vastu or Feng Shui to create a balanced and harmonious home.

9. Practice Mindfulness and Self-Awareness: Cultivate mindfulness and self-awareness in your daily life. Pay attention to your thoughts, emotions, and physical sensations. Take moments throughout the day to pause, breathe, and check in with yourself. This practice allows you to make conscious choices aligned with your well-being.

10. Seek Guidance: If you are new to Ayurveda, consider seeking guidance from an Ayurvedic practitioner or attending workshops and classes to deepen your understanding and practice. A practitioner can provide personalized recommendations based on your unique constitution and health goals.

Remember, Ayurveda is a journey of self-discovery and transformation. Start by incorporating small changes into your daily routine and gradually build upon them. Listen to your body, honor its needs, and adapt your practices as you gain deeper insights into your own well-being. By integrating Ayurvedic wisdom into your life, you can experience enhanced vitality, balance, and overall wellness.

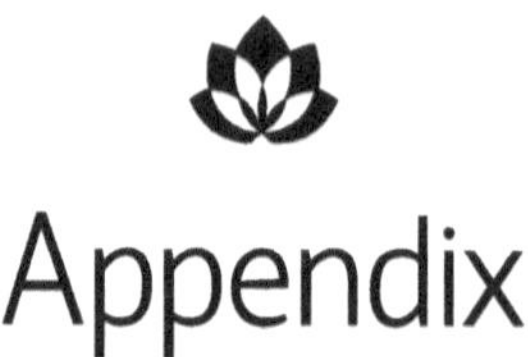

Appendix

- Resources for further exploration and study
- Glossary of Ayurvedic terms
- Sample Ayurvedic recipes and meal plans
- Ayurvedic self-assessment tools and quizzes

  - Dosha Questionnaire (To Assess Prakriti / Bodytype)
  - Ayurvedic Lifestyle Assessment
  - Food and Digestion Quiz
  - Ayurvedic Emotional Wellness Inventory

Resources for Further Exploration and Study of Ayurveda

1. Books:
- "The Complete Book of Ayurvedic Home Remedies" by Vasant Lad
- "Ayurveda: The Science of Self-Healing" by Dr. Vasant Lad
    - "The Perfect Health" by Deepak Chopra
- "Prakriti: Your Ayurvedic Constitution" by Dr. Robert E. Svoboda
- "Ayurvedic Healing: A Comprehensive Guide" by Dr. David Frawley
- "Ayurveda: Secrets of Healing" by Maya Tiwari
    2. Online Courses and Programs:
- Ayurveda Online Courses by the Ayurvedic Institute (ayurveda.com)
- Ayurveda Courses and Workshops by the Chopra Center (chopra.com)
- Ayurveda Foundations Course by the California College of Ayurveda (ayurvedacollege.com)
    3. Ayurvedic Practitioners and Teachers:
- Seek guidance from certified Ayurvedic practitioners and teachers in your

area. They can provide personalized recommendations and guidance based on your specific needs.

4. Ayurvedic Retreats and Workshops:
- Participate in Ayurvedic retreats or workshops that offer immersive experiences and practical knowledge of Ayurveda. Look for reputable retreat centers or wellness centers that specialize in Ayurvedic practices.

5. Ayurvedic Organizations and Journals:
- International Association of Ayurveda (ayurved-int.com)
- National Ayurvedic Medical Association (ayurvedanama.org)
- Ayurveda Journal of Health (ayurvedajournal.org)

6. Online Resources:
- Easy Ayurveda (easyayurveda.com): A wealth of information on Ayurveda for both general public and Ayurveda professionals
- Banyan Botanicals (banyanbotanicals.com): Offers a wealth of information on Ayurvedic herbs, recipes, and lifestyle practices.
- Ayurveda.com: Provides resources, articles, and information on Ayurvedic principles and practices.
- Ayurvedic Institute (ayurveda.com): Features resources, articles, and educational materials on Ayurveda.

7. Ayurvedic Clinics and Wellness Centers:
- Visit Ayurvedic clinics and wellness centers that offer consultations, treatments, and educational programs. These centers can provide a holistic approach to Ayurvedic healing.

8. Ayurvedic Conferences and Events:
- Attend Ayurvedic conferences, seminars, and workshops to deepen your understanding and connect with experts in the field. These events often feature renowned Ayurvedic practitioners, researchers, and educators.

Remember, Ayurveda is a vast and ancient system of knowledge. Exploring and studying Ayurveda is a lifelong journey, and it is important to approach it with an open mind and a commitment to self-discovery. Choose resources and teachers that resonate with you and align with your goals and values. Embrace Ayurveda as a transformative path towards holistic well-being and a deeper connection with yourself and the world around you.

Glossary of Ayurvedic Terms

Ayurveda: The ancient holistic system of medicine from India, focusing on maintaining health and preventing disease through balance and harmony of the mind, body, and spirit.

Dosha: The three bioenergetic forces or constitutions in Ayurveda—Vata, Pitta, and Kapha—that govern the physiological and psychological aspects of an individual.

Prakriti: The unique individual constitution determined by the dominant dosha(s) present at the time of conception, which influences physical and mental characteristics.

Vata: The dosha associated with the elements of air and space. It governs movement, creativity, and the nervous system.

Pitta: The dosha associated with the elements of fire and water. It governs metabolism, digestion, and transformation.

Kapha: The dosha associated with the elements of earth and water. It governs stability, structure, and lubrication.

Agni: The digestive fire responsible for the digestion and assimilation of food, as well as the transformation of thoughts, emotions, and experiences.

Dhatu: The seven tissue layers in the body—plasma, blood, muscle, fat, bone, bone marrow, and reproductive tissue—formed sequentially from food and processed by Agni.

Srotas: The channels or systems responsible for the transportation of nutrients, waste, and information throughout the body.

Ojas: The vital essence of life, representing the body's immunity, vitality, and strength.

Ama: The toxic waste or undigested material that accumulates in the body due to incomplete digestion and metabolic imbalances.

Prana: The life force or vital energy that flows through the body, responsible for sustaining all bodily functions.

Sattva: The quality of purity, clarity, and harmony. It represents a state of balanced mind, calmness, and contentment.

Rajas: The quality of activity, movement, and restlessness. It represents a state of passion, ambition, and desires.

Tamas: The quality of inertia, darkness, and heaviness. It represents a state of lethargy, ignorance, and stagnation.

Rasayana: The rejuvenation and longevity practices in Ayurveda, aimed at preserving youthfulness, vitality, and overall well-being.

Panchakarma: The Ayurvedic detoxification and purification therapies that remove toxins, restore balance, and rejuvenate the body.

Abhyanga: The Ayurvedic self-massage technique using warm herbal oils to nourish the body, promote circulation, and release tension.

Neti: The nasal cleansing practice using warm saline water to clear the nasal passages and promote respiratory health.

Nasya: The administration of medicated oils or herbal powders through the nasal passages to support nasal health and balance the doshas.

Dinacharya: The daily routine practices in Ayurveda, including waking up early, tongue scraping, oil pulling, bathing, and other self-care rituals.

Ritucharya: The seasonal routine practices that help the body adapt to the changes in weather and maintain balance throughout the year.

Rasas: The six tastes—sweet, sour, salty, bitter, pungent, and astringent—representing different combinations of the five elements and their effects on the doshas and body.

Sattvic Diet: A pure and balanced diet consisting of fresh, organic, vegetarian foods that promote clarity, peace, and spiritual growth.

Vata-Pacifying Diet: A diet that includes warm, grounding, and nourishing foods to balance Vata dosha's cold, dry, and light qualities.

Pitta-Pacifying Diet: A diet that includes cooling, soothing, and hydrating foods to balance Pitta dosha's hot, sharp, and intense qualities.

Kapha-Pacifying Diet: A diet that includes light, warm, and stimulating foods to balance Kapha dosha's heavy, cold, and stagnant qualities.

Herbs: Plant-based medicines and remedies used in Ayurveda to support healing, balance the doshas, and promote overall well-being.

Manas: The mind, encompassing thoughts, emotions, and mental processes.

Ahara: The intake of food, including both physical and energetic aspects of nourishment.

Vihara: Lifestyle practices and habits that support overall well-being, including sleep, exercise, and daily routines.

Sadhana: Spiritual practices or disciplines aimed at personal growth, self-realization, and inner transformation.

Sadhaka Pitta: Subdosha of Pitta related to emotions, perception, and the heart.

Ojas-tejas-shakti: The subtle energies responsible for immunity, radiance, and inner strength.

Sthira: The quality of stability, steadiness, and groundedness.

Sukha: The quality of ease, happiness, and contentment.

Dukha: The quality of suffering, pain, or discomfort.

Swastha: The state of optimal health and well-being.

Vishama Agni: Irregular or variable digestive fire.

Sama Agni: Balanced and healthy digestive fire.

Viruddha Ahara: Incompatible food combinations that can disrupt digestion and lead to imbalances.

Srotodushti: Impairment or imbalance of the channels or systems in the body.

Satmya: The principle of individual adaptability and tolerance to specific foods, climates, and environments.

Marma Points: Vital energy points in the body that are sensitive and can be stimulated for therapeutic purposes.

Pulse Diagnosis: The practice of assessing the qualities of the pulse to gather information about the dosha imbalances and overall health.

Jatharagni: The digestive fire located in the stomach responsible for breaking down food.

Anupana: Carrier substances used to enhance the efficacy of herbs or medicines.

Nidra: The state of sleep or restful slumber.

Srotamsi: The microchannels or pathways that transport nutrients and waste products within the body.

Svedana: The practice of therapeutic sweating, which helps eliminate toxins and balance the doshas.

Basti: A therapeutic enema treatment to cleanse and rejuvenate the colon.

Garshana: Dry brushing technique to stimulate circulation and lymphatic flow.

Udvartana: Ayurvedic herbal powder massage for exfoliation and detoxification.

Gandusha: Oil pulling or swishing warm oil in the mouth for oral health.

Kavala: Gargling with herbal decoctions or oils for oral hygiene.

Vamana: Therapeutic vomiting or induced emesis to eliminate toxins from the body.

Raktamokshana: Bloodletting or therapeutic blood cleansing technique.

Shirodhara: Pouring a continuous stream of warm oil over the forehead to calm the mind and promote relaxation.

Ayurvedic Terms for Common Conditions:

- Agni Mandya: Weak digestion
- Ama Visha: Toxic accumulation
- Prana Vata: Subdosha of Vata related to respiration and sensory perception
- Ranjaka Pitta: Subdosha of Pitta responsible for liver function and blood

quality
- Meda Dhatu: The fat tissue
- Asthi Dhatu: The bone tissue
- Majja Dhatu: The bone marrow and nervous tissue
- Shukra Dhatu: The reproductive tissue
   Note: This glossary provides a brief overview of Ayurvedic terms. For a comprehensive understanding, it is recommended to study Ayurveda under the guidance of qualified practitioners or refer to authoritative Ayurvedic texts.

Sample Ayurvedic Recipes and Meal Plans

1. Vata-Pacifying Meal Plan:
- Breakfast: Warm oatmeal with cooked apples, cinnamon, and a sprinkle of chopped almonds.
- Lunch: Mung bean soup with steamed vegetables and a side of quinoa.
- Snack: Roasted pumpkin seeds with a sprinkle of turmeric and black pepper.
- Dinner: Baked salmon with roasted sweet potatoes and steamed broccoli.
- Evening Drink: Boiled and cooled ginger tea with a dash of honey.
   2. Pitta-Pacifying Meal Plan:
- Breakfast: Cooling smoothie with coconut water, cucumber, mint, and a pinch of cardamom.
- Lunch: Quinoa salad with mixed greens, cherry tomatoes, avocado, and a drizzle of lemon-tahini dressing.
- Snack: Sliced watermelon or a cooling fruit salad.
- Dinner: Grilled tofu with sautéed zucchini and brown rice.
- Evening Drink: Aloe vera juice or a refreshing mint-infused water.
   3. Kapha-Pacifying Meal Plan:
- Breakfast: Warm spiced quinoa porridge with grated ginger, cinnamon, and chopped dates.
- Lunch: Lentil soup with lots of vegetables and a squeeze of lemon.
- Snack: Sliced apples with a sprinkle of cinnamon and a small handful of walnuts.
- Dinner: Stir-fried vegetables with tofu or lean chicken breast and a side of quinoa.
- Evening Drink: Warm ginger tea with a squeeze of lemon and a dash of cayenne pepper.

Note: The meal plans provided are general guidelines. It is important to tailor them to your individual needs and consult with a qualified Ayurvedic practitioner for personalized recommendations.

Sample Ayurvedic Recipes:

1. Ayurvedic Kitchari:

Ingredients:

- 1/2 cup basmati rice
- 1/2 cup split yellow mung beans
- 1 tablespoon ghee
- 1 teaspoon cumin seeds
- 1 teaspoon grated ginger
- 1/2 teaspoon turmeric powder
- 4 cups water
- Salt to taste
- Fresh cilantro for garnish

Instructions:

1. Wash the rice and mung beans together until the water runs clear.
2. In a large pot, heat the ghee and add the cumin seeds. Sauté until fragrant.
3. Add the grated ginger, turmeric powder, rice, and mung beans. Stir well.
4. Add water and bring to a boil. Reduce heat, cover, and simmer for about 30-40 minutes until the grains are cooked and the mixture becomes porridge-like.
5. Season with salt to taste. Garnish with fresh cilantro and serve warm.

2. Golden Milk:

Ingredients:

- 1 cup almond milk (or any non-dairy milk)
- 1 teaspoon turmeric powder
- 1/2 teaspoon cinnamon powder
- 1/4 teaspoon ginger powder
- Pinch of black pepper
- 1 teaspoon honey (optional- don't add when it's hot)

Instructions:

1. In a small saucepan, heat the almond milk over low heat.
2. Add turmeric, cinnamon, ginger, and black pepper. Whisk well to combine.
3. Simmer for about 5 minutes, stirring occasionally.
4. Remove from heat and add honey after cooling, if desired.
5. Pour into a mug and enjoy warm.

3. Triphala Tea:

Ingredients:

- 1 teaspoon Triphala powder
- 2 cups water
- Honey (optional)

Instructions:

1. Bring the water to a boil in a small saucepan.
2. Add the Triphala powder to the boiling water.
3. Reduce the heat and let it simmer for 10 minutes.
4. Strain the tea into a cup.
5. Add honey after cooling down, if desired, and enjoy.

4. Ayurvedic Green Smoothie:

Ingredients:

- 1 cup spinach
- 1 small cucumber
- 1 ripe banana
- 1 tablespoon almond butter
- 1 teaspoon chia seeds
- 1 cup coconut water
- 1/2 teaspoon spirulina powder

Instructions:

1. Place all the ingredients in a blender.
2. Blend until smooth and creamy.
3. Pour into a glass and enjoy immediately.

5. Masoor Dal Soup:

Ingredients:

- 1 cup masoor dal (red lentils)
- 4 cups water
- 1 tablespoon ghee
- 1 teaspoon cumin seeds
- 1 teaspoon grated ginger
- 1/2 teaspoon turmeric powder
- 1/2 teaspoon coriander powder
- Salt to taste
- Fresh cilantro for garnish

Instructions:

1. Wash the masoor dal until the water runs clear.
2. In a large pot, heat the ghee and add the cumin seeds. Sauté until fragrant.

3. Add the grated ginger, turmeric powder, coriander powder, and washed masoor dal. Stir well.

4. Add water and bring to a boil. Reduce heat, cover, and simmer for about 20-25 minutes until the lentils are soft and cooked.

5. Season with salt to taste. Garnish with fresh cilantro and serve hot.

Feel free to explore Ayurvedic cookbooks, online resources, and consult with an Ayurvedic practitioner for more recipes that align with your dosha and health goals. Enjoy the journey of nourishing your body and mind through Ayurvedic cooking!

Remember to use organic and fresh ingredients whenever possible and adjust the recipes based on your dosha and specific dietary requirements. These recipes are a starting point, and you can experiment with different Ayurvedic herbs, spices, and ingredients to create meals that suit your taste preferences and health needs.

Ayurveda Tools and Quizzes

Dosha Questionnaire (To Assess Prakriti / Bodytype)

Instructions:

This Dosha Questionnaire is designed to help you gain insights into your unique constitution and determine your dominant dosha(s) according to Ayurvedic principles. Please answer the following questions to the best of your ability. Be honest and choose the response that most accurately reflects your tendencies and characteristics. Remember, this questionnaire is not a definitive diagnosis, but rather a tool to provide you with a general understanding of your dosha composition. Consult with an Ayurvedic practitioner for a more accurate assessment.

Disclaimer:

The Dosha Questionnaire is not a substitute for professional medical advice, diagnosis, or treatment. It is intended for educational purposes only. The results of this questionnaire should not be used to self-diagnose or self-treat any health condition. If you have any concerns about your health, it is recommended to seek guidance from a qualified healthcare professional.

Questionnaire:

Physical Characteristics:

1. What is your body frame like?

a) Thin and slender

b) Moderate, neither too thin nor too heavy

c) Solid and well-built

2. How is your skin texture?

a) Dry and rough

b) Soft and smooth

c) Oily and prone to breakouts

3. How would you describe your hair?

a) Dry and brittle

b) Fine and lustrous

c) Thick and oily

4. What is your typical body temperature?

a) Cold hands and feet, overall low body temperature

b) Moderate body temperature

c) Warm hands and feet, overall high body temperature

5. How would you describe your appetite?

a) Variable, sometimes weak

b) Strong and steady

c) Intense and quick to feel hungry

Mental and Emotional Tendencies:

6. How do you generally respond to stress?

a) Worried and anxious

b) Ambitious and driven

c) Irritable and impatient

7. How would you describe your energy levels throughout the day?

a) Low and easily fatigued

b) Moderate and steady

c) High and fluctuating

8. What is your usual sleep pattern?

a) Light sleeper, difficulty falling asleep

b) Moderate sleeper, generally sound sleep

c) Deep sleeper, tendency to oversleep

9. How do you handle change and new experiences?

a) Prefer routine and resist change

b) Adapt well to change

c) Embrace change and seek new experiences

10. How would you describe your memory and learning abilities?
a) Quick to forget, tendency to be scattered
b) Average memory and learning abilities
c) Sharp memory, quick to grasp new concepts
Assessment:
For each question, assign the following points based on your response:
a) -1 point
b) 0 points
c) +1 point
Add up the total points for each dosha:
Vata: ________
Pitta: ________
Kapha: ________
Interpretation:
- If your Vata score is highest, you have a dominant Vata constitution.
- If your Pitta score is highest, you have a dominant Pitta constitution.
- If your Kapha score is highest, you have a dominant Kapha constitution.
- If you have similar scores for two doshas, you may have a dual dosha constitution (e.g., Vata-Pitta, Pitta-Kapha, Vata-Kapha).
- If all three doshas have equal scores, you may have a Tridoshic constitution.

Note: This questionnaire provides a general assessment and should be used as a starting point to understand your dosha composition. For a more accurate assessment and personalized recommendations, consult with an Ayurvedic practitioner.

Remember, Ayurveda is a holistic system, and a comprehensive evaluation of your physical, mental, and emotional state is necessary for a complete understanding of your constitution.

Disclaimer:
Please consult with a qualified Ayurvedic practitioner or healthcare professional for a more accurate assessment and personalized guidance. The Dosha Questionnaire is not intended to diagnose or treat any health condition. The results should be used as a tool for self-exploration and education about Ayurveda.

Ayurvedic Lifestyle Assessment

Instructions:

The Ayurvedic Lifestyle Assessment is a self-assessment tool designed to help you evaluate your daily routines and lifestyle habits in order to gain insights into any imbalances and make practical changes for a more balanced and harmonious life according to Ayurvedic principles. Please answer the following questions honestly and choose the response that best reflects your current habits and routines. The assessment is intended to provide general guidance and suggestions, but for a more personalized approach, it is recommended to consult with an Ayurvedic practitioner.

Disclaimer:

The Ayurvedic Lifestyle Assessment is not a substitute for professional medical advice, diagnosis, or treatment. It is intended for educational purposes only. The results of this assessment should not be used to self-diagnose or self-treat any health condition. If you have any concerns about your health, it is recommended to seek guidance from a qualified healthcare professional.

Instructions for Use:

1. Read each question carefully and choose the response that best applies to you.

2. Score yourself according to the provided options.

3. Total your scores for each section and refer to the interpretation guide below.

4. Use the results to identify areas where you may need to make adjustments in your lifestyle.

Ayurvedic Lifestyle Assessment:

1. Waking Routine:

a) I wake up feeling refreshed and energized. (+2)

b) I often wake up feeling groggy or tired. (+1)

c) I struggle to wake up and feel lethargic. (0)

2. Sleep Routine:

a) I consistently get 7-8 hours of quality sleep. (+2)

b) I sometimes have difficulty falling asleep or staying asleep. (+1)

c) I frequently have trouble sleeping and wake up feeling unrested. (0)

3. Meal Times:

a) I have regular meal times and eat mindfully. (+2)

b) I sometimes skip meals or eat irregularly. (+1)

c) I often eat on-the-go or have erratic eating habits. (0)

4. Diet:

a) I eat a balanced diet of fresh, whole foods. (+2)

b) I occasionally indulge in processed or unhealthy foods. (+1)

c) I frequently rely on processed or unhealthy foods. (0)

5. Exercise:

a) I engage in regular exercise or physical activity. (+2)

b) I exercise sporadically or inconsistently. (+1)

c) I lead a sedentary lifestyle with minimal physical activity. (0)

6. Stress Levels:

a) I effectively manage stress and feel calm and balanced. (+2)

b) I experience occasional stress but can manage it reasonably well. (+1)

c) I often feel overwhelmed and struggle with managing stress. (0)

7. Self-Care:

a) I prioritize self-care and engage in regular relaxation practices. (+2)

b) I occasionally make time for self-care but could do more. (+1)

c) I rarely prioritize self-care and often neglect my own needs. (0)

Assessment:

Total your scores for each section and refer to the interpretation guide below:

Waking Routine:

- Score 4-6: Your waking routine is in alignment with Ayurvedic principles.

- Score 2-3: There may be some room for improvement in your waking routine.

- Score 0-1: Your waking routine may require significant adjustments for balance.

Sleep Routine:

- Score 4-6: Your sleep routine is in alignment with Ayurvedic principles.

- Score 2-3: There may be some room for improvement in your sleep routine.

- Score 0-1: Your sleep routine may require significant adjustments for balance.

Meal Times:

- Score 4-6: Your meal times are in alignment with Ayurvedic principles.

- Score 2-3: There may be some room for improvement in your meal times.

- Score 0-1: Your meal times may require significant adjustments for balance.

Diet:

- Score 4-6: Your diet is in alignment with Ayurvedic principles.

- Score 2-3: There may be some room for improvement in your diet.
- Score 0-1: Your diet may require significant adjustments for balance.

Exercise:
- Score 4-6: Your exercise routine is in alignment with Ayurvedic principles.
- Score 2-3: There may be some room for improvement in your exercise routine.
- Score 0-1: Your exercise routine may require significant adjustments for balance.

Stress Levels:
- Score 4-6: Your stress levels are in alignment with Ayurvedic principles.
- Score 2-3: There may be some room for improvement in managing your stress.
- Score 0-1: Your stress levels may require significant adjustments for balance.

Self-Care:
- Score 4-6: Your self-care practices are in alignment with Ayurvedic principles.
- Score 2-3: There may be some room for improvement in your self-care practices.
- Score 0-1: Your self-care practices may require significant adjustments for balance.

Please note that this self-assessment is a general guideline and not a substitute for personalized advice from an Ayurvedic practitioner. Use the results to identify areas where you can make positive changes to align with Ayurvedic principles and consult with a qualified practitioner for a more comprehensive evaluation and personalized recommendations.

Food and Digestion Quiz

Instructions:
The Food and Digestion Quiz is designed to help you assess your eating habits, food preferences, and digestive patterns. Please answer the following questions honestly and choose the response that best reflects your current situation. The quiz aims to provide insights into your digestion and offer recommendations for optimizing your diet and enhancing overall digestive well-being. However, for personalized advice, it is recommended to consult with an Ayurvedic practitioner or healthcare professional.

Disclaimer:

The Food and Digestion Quiz is not intended to diagnose or treat any medical condition. It is for informational purposes only and should not replace professional medical advice. The quiz results should be used as a tool for self-assessment and education about Ayurvedic principles. If you have specific health concerns or dietary restrictions, it is recommended to seek guidance from a qualified healthcare professional.

Instructions for Use:

1. Read each question carefully and choose the response that best applies to you.

2. Score yourself according to the provided options.

3. Total your scores for each section and refer to the interpretation guide below.

4. Use the results to identify areas for improvement in your diet and digestion.

Food and Digestion Quiz:

1. How would you describe your appetite?

a) Strong and consistent.

b) Varies from day to day.

c) Weak or irregular.

2. Do you experience any food cravings?

a) Rarely or never.

b) Occasionally, but not frequently.

c) Frequently or consistently.

3. How do you feel after eating a meal?

a) Satisfied and energized.

b) Sometimes bloated or heavy.

c) Often uncomfortable or lethargic.

4. Do you experience any digestive issues such as bloating, gas, or indigestion?

a) Rarely or never.

b) Occasionally, but not frequently.

c) Frequently or consistently.

5. How do you react to spicy or hot foods?

a) I enjoy and tolerate them well.

b) I can handle them in moderation.

c) I find them difficult to digest.

6. Do you have any specific food allergies or sensitivities?
a) No, I have no known allergies or sensitivities.
b) Yes, I have mild allergies or sensitivities.
c) Yes, I have significant allergies or sensitivities.

7. How often do you consume processed or packaged foods?
a) Rarely or never.
b) Occasionally, but not frequently.
c) Frequently or consistently.

Assessment:

Total your scores for each section and refer to the interpretation guide below:

Appetite:
- Score 7-10: Your appetite is generally strong and consistent.
- Score 4-6: Your appetite varies, and it may be helpful to establish regular eating times.
- Score 0-3: Your appetite is weak or irregular, and it may be beneficial to work on improving it.

Food Cravings:
- Score 7-10: You experience few cravings, indicating a balanced diet.
- Score 4-6: You have occasional cravings, which may be managed with mindful eating.
- Score 0-3: You have frequent cravings, suggesting potential imbalances in your diet.

Digestion:
- Score 7-10: Your digestion is generally strong, and you experience minimal discomfort.
- Score 4-6: You occasionally experience digestive issues, indicating the need for mindful eating practices.
- Score 0-3: You frequently experience digestive issues, suggesting imbalances that may require attention.

Reactions to Spicy Foods:
- Score 7-10: You tolerate spicy foods well and enjoy them in moderation.
- Score 4-6: You have a moderate tolerance for spicy foods, and it may be beneficial to consume them in moderation.
- Score 0-3: You struggle with digesting spicy foods, and it may be best to avoid or minimize their consumption.

Food Allergies/Sensitivities:
- Score 7-10: You have no known allergies or sensitivities.

- Score 4-6: You have mild allergies or sensitivities, and it may be beneficial to avoid trigger foods.
- Score 0-3: You have significant allergies or sensitivities, and it is important to avoid trigger foods.

Processed/Packaged Foods:
- Score 7-10: You rarely consume processed or packaged foods, prioritizing whole and fresh ingredients.
- Score 4-6: You occasionally consume processed or packaged foods, and it may be beneficial to reduce their intake.
- Score 0-3: You frequently consume processed or packaged foods, and it is recommended to prioritize whole foods for better digestion and health.

Remember, this quiz is a general guide and not a substitute for professional advice. Use the results to gain insights into your eating habits and digestive patterns. If you have specific dietary concerns or health conditions, it is recommended to consult with an Ayurvedic practitioner or healthcare professional for personalized recommendations.

Ayurvedic Emotional Wellness Inventory

Instructions:
The Ayurvedic Emotional Wellness Inventory is designed to assess your emotional well-being and stress levels. This tool will provide insights into your ability to manage stress, cope with emotions, and maintain emotional balance. Please answer the following questions honestly and choose the response that best reflects your current situation. The inventory aims to help you identify areas for improvement and offer suggestions for incorporating Ayurvedic practices such as meditation, breathing exercises, and self-care rituals into your daily routine. It is important to note that this inventory does not replace professional mental health advice. If you are experiencing severe emotional distress or have mental health concerns, it is recommended to seek guidance from a qualified healthcare professional.

Disclaimer:
The Ayurvedic Emotional Wellness Inventory is not intended to diagnose or treat any mental health condition. It is for informational purposes only and should not replace professional mental health advice. The inventory results should be used as a tool for self-assessment and education about Ayurvedic principles. If you have specific mental health concerns, it is recommended to consult with a mental health professional or Ayurvedic practitioner for

personalized guidance.

Instructions for Use:

1. Read each question carefully and choose the response that best applies to you.

2. Score yourself according to the provided options.

3. Total your scores for each section and refer to the interpretation guide below.

4. Use the results to identify areas for improvement in your emotional well-being.

Ayurvedic Emotional Wellness Inventory:

1. How often do you experience stress?

a) Rarely or never.

b) Occasionally.

c) Frequently or consistently.

2. How well do you cope with stress?

a) I manage stress effectively and have healthy coping mechanisms.

b) I can cope with stress to some extent, but there is room for improvement.

c) I struggle to cope with stress and often feel overwhelmed.

3. How do you handle your emotions?

a) I can acknowledge and express my emotions in a healthy way.

b) I sometimes struggle to manage my emotions but make an effort to work through them.

c) I find it challenging to handle my emotions, and they often impact my well-being.

4. How often do you practice relaxation techniques such as meditation or deep breathing?

a) Regularly, I have a consistent practice.

b) Occasionally, but I recognize the benefits and would like to incorporate it more.

c) Rarely or never, I have difficulty finding time or motivation for relaxation practices.

5. How well do you prioritize self-care and self-nurturing activities?

a) I prioritize self-care and regularly engage in activities that support my well-being.

b) I make an effort to practice self-care, but there is room for improvement.

c) I struggle to prioritize self-care and often neglect my own needs.

6. How balanced do you feel emotionally on a day-to-day basis?

a) I generally feel emotionally balanced and resilient.

b) I experience emotional ups and downs but can find stability with effort.

c) I often feel emotionally imbalanced and find it challenging to regain equilibrium.

Assessment:

Total your scores for each section and refer to the interpretation guide below:

Stress Level:

- Score 7-10: You experience minimal stress in your life.

- Score 4-6: You experience moderate levels of stress that can be managed with stress-reducing techniques.

- Score 0-3: You experience high levels of stress and may benefit from incorporating more stress-management practices into your routine.

Coping with Stress:

- Score 7-10: You have effective coping mechanisms and manage stress well.

- Score 4-6: You have some coping strategies, but there is room for improvement.

- Score 0-3: You struggle to cope with stress and may benefit from learning additional techniques for managing stress.

Emotional Regulation:

- Score 7-10: You have healthy emotional regulation skills and can handle emotions effectively.

- Score 4-6: You have some emotional regulation skills, but there is room for improvement.

- Score 0-3: You find it challenging to manage emotions, and they often impact your well-being.

Relaxation Practices:

- Score 7-10: You have a regular practice of relaxation techniques, which contributes to your emotional well-being.

- Score 4-6: You occasionally engage in relaxation practices but would benefit from making them a more consistent part of your routine.

- Score 0-3: You rarely or never engage in relaxation practices, and incorporating them into your routine can greatly benefit your emotional well-being.

Self-Care:

- Score 7-10: You prioritize self-care and actively engage in nurturing activities that support your well-being.

- Score 4-6: You make some effort to practice self-care, but there is room for improvement.

- Score 0-3: You struggle to prioritize self-care and often neglect your own needs.

Emotional Balance:

- Score 7-10: You generally feel emotionally balanced and resilient.

- Score 4-6: You experience emotional ups and downs but can find stability with effort.

- Score 0-3: You often feel emotionally imbalanced and find it challenging to regain equilibrium.

Remember, this inventory is a tool for self-assessment and general guidance. Use the results to gain insights into your emotional well-being and consider incorporating Ayurvedic practices to enhance your overall emotional wellness. If you have specific mental health concerns, it is recommended to seek guidance from a qualified mental health professional or Ayurvedic practitioner.

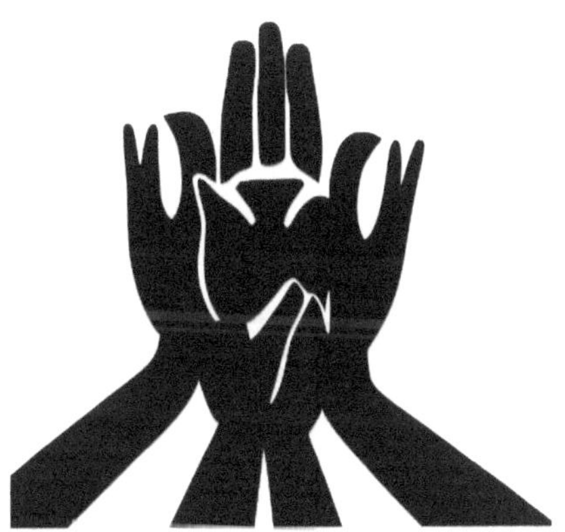

Thank You | Namaste

Disclaimer: The information in this book is intended for educational purposes only and should not replace professional medical advice. Consult a qualified Ayurvedic practitioner or healthcare provider before making any changes to your health routine.